ER/ICU Meds Made Easy

Callie Parker

Copyright

Copyright © 2025 by Callie Parker

All rights reserved.

No portion of this book may be reproduced in any form without written permission from the publisher or author, except as permitted by U.S. copyright law.

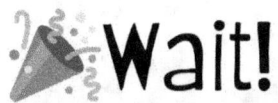 **Wait!** Before You Dive In... Grab Your FREE Nursing Study Survival Kit!

Nursing school is no joke—that's why MadeEasy.Academy is committed to sending the ladder back down and rescuing those of you in the trenches!

Ready to study smarter, not harder? We've got exactly what you need.

Your FREE NCLEX in My Sleep Bundle Includes:

✅ Who's Dying First? The Prioritization Playbook: Because patient safety is kind of a big deal. 😅
✅ Flashcard Frenzy: Memorize or Die Trying: Pre-made Anki cards to save your sanity.
✅ WTF Does This Lab Value Mean? Cheat Sheet: No more second-guessing normal vs. "oh sh*t" levels.
✅ NCLEX Mnemonics That Stick (Like Tape on an IV Line): Memory hacks you'll actually remember.
✅ Med Math Without the Mental Breakdown: Because no one wants to commit a dosage error. 😬

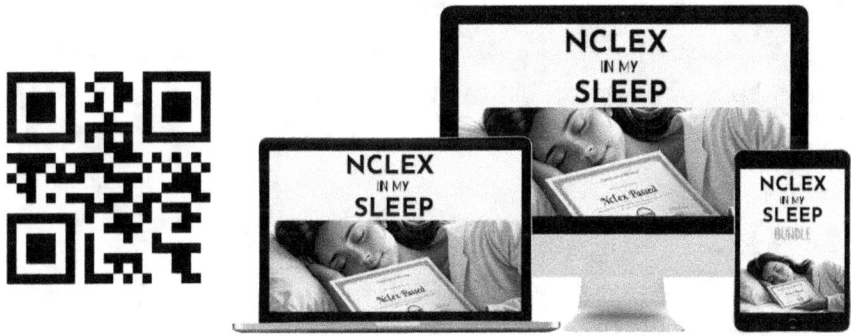

Head over to MadeEasy.Academy to grab your bundle. Let's turn nursing school stress into success!

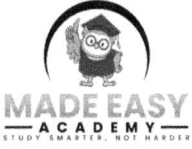

But that's not all...
🎁 BONUS 🎁

Your Bundle Includes an Exclusive 50% OFF Discount Code for your next course at Made Easy Academy
(Launching June 1!)

At <u>MadeEasy.Academy</u> we don't just simplify nursing—we transform it into an effortless, memorable study process.

For each topic, you'll follow our step by step success guide:

 Step 1. Grab your cheat sheet: All key points, zero fluff.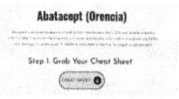

 Step 2. Read your mnemonic poem: Clever rhymes to make information stick.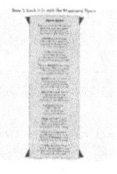

 Step 3. Take your fill-in-the-blank quiz: Test your recall without the overwhelm.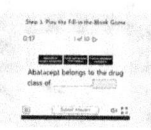

 Step 4. Complete your NCLEX challenge: Realistic practice questions with clear rationales.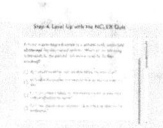

 Step 5. Walk Into the NCLEX Like a Boss: Confident, prepared, and ready to pass.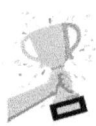

Right now, we're laser-focused on Pharmacology, but we'll soon expand into other crucial nursing topics! Have a topic you want us to cover next? Shoot us an email at hello@madeeasy.academy—we've got you!

Table of Contents

Made Easy: Why and How
Pharmacology Mind Maps
Pharmacology Mind Map Template
Neurotransmitters & Their Functions Chart
Pharmacology Mnemonics

Part I
Analgesics, Antipyretics & Sedation 1
   Analgesics, Antipyretics & Sedation 3
   Acetaminophen (Tylenol) 5
   Dexamethasone (Decadron) 6
   Diazepam (Valium) 7
   Dexmedetomidine (Precedex) 8
   Diphenhydramine (Benadryl) 9
   Etomidate (Amidate) 10
   Fentanyl (Sublimaze) 11
   Hydromorphone (Dilaudid) 12
   Ibuprofen (Advil, Motrin) 13
   Ketamine (Ketalar) 14
   Ketorolac (Toradol) 15
   Lidocaine (Xylocaine) 16
   Lorazepam (Ativan) 17
   Midazolam (Versed) 18
   Morphine 19
   Oxycodone (OxyContin, Roxicodone) 20
   Propofol (Diprivan) 21

Part II
Cardiovascular & Hemodynamic Support 23
   Adenosine (Adenocard) 25
   Albumin (Albuminar, Albutein) 26
   Amiodarone (Cordarone, Pacerone) 27
   Angiotensin II (Giapreza) 28
   Aspirin (ASA) 29
   Atropine (Atropen) 30
   Clevidipine (Cleviprex) 31
   Diltiazem (Cardizem) 32
   Digoxin (Lanoxin) 33
   Dobutamine 34
   Dopamine (Intropin) 35

Ephedrine	36
Epinephrine (Adrenalin)	37
Esmolol (Brevibloc)	38
Hydralazine (Apresoline)	39
Isoproterenol (Isuprel)	40
Isosorbide Dinitrate	41
Levosimendan	42
Metoprolol (Lopressor)	43
Milrinone (Primacor)	44
Nicardipine (Cardene)	45
Nimodipine	46
Nitroglycerin (Nitrostat, Tridil)	47
Nitroprusside (Nipride)	48
Norepinephrine (Levophed)	49
Phenylephrine (Neo-Synephrine)	50
Phentolamine	51
Procainamide (Pronestyl)	52
Propranolol (Inderal)	53
Ranolazine (Ranexa)	54
Vasopressin (Pitressin)	55
Verapamil (Calan, Isoptin)	56

Part III
Thrombolytics, Anticoagulants & Reversal Agents 57

Alteplase (Activase)	59
Andexanet Alfa	60
Argatroban	61
Bivalirudin	62
Clopidogrel (Plavix)	63
Enalapril (Vasotec)	64
Enoxaparin (Lovenox)	65
Eptifibatide (Integrilin)	66
Heparin	67
Idarucizumab (Praxbind)	68
Protamine Sulfate	69
Reteplase (Retavase)	70
Tenecteplase (TNKase)	71
Ticagrelor (Brilinta)	72
Tirofiban (Aggrastat)	73
Tranexamic Acid (Cyklokapron)	74
Warfarin (Coumadin)	75

Part IV
Neurologic & Seizure Management 77

Dantrolene (Dantrium)	79

Fosphenytoin (Cerebyx) 80
Lacosamide (Vimpat) 81
Levetiracetam (Keppra) 82
Nalmefene 83
Naloxone (Narcan) 84
Neostigmine 85
Phenytoin (Dilantin) 86
Phenobarbital 87
Propafenone (Rythmol) 88
Valproic Acid (Depakote) 89

Part V
Reversal Agents & Toxicology 91
Acetylcysteine (Mucomyst) 93
Andexanet Alfa 94
Digoxin Immune Fab (DigiFab) 95
Flumazenil (Romazicon) 96
Hydroxycobalamin 97
Idarucizumab (Praxbind) 98
Intralipid 99
Methylene Blue 100
Sodium Bicarbonate 101

Part VI
Antibiotics & Antimicrobials 103
Azithromycin (Zithromax) 105
Ceftriaxone (Rocephin) 106
Ciprofloxacin (Cipro) 107
Metronidazole (Flagyl) 108
Meropenem 109
Piperacillin-Tazobactam (Zosyn) 110
Vancomycin (Vancocin) 111

Part VII
GI, Endocrine & Electrolyte Support 113
Desmopressin (DDAVP, Nocdurna, Stimate) 115
Dextrose 50% (D50) 116
Esomeprazole (Nexium) 117
Famotidine (Pepcid) 118
Glucagon (GlucaGen) 119
Insulin Regular (Humulin R, Novolin R) 120
Metoclopramide (Reglan) 121
Omeprazole (Prilosec) 122
Octreotide (Sandostatin) 123
Pantoprazole (Protonix) 124

Potassium Chloride (K-Dur, Klor-Con) 125
  Prednisone 126
  Sodium Polystyrene Sulfonate (Kayexalate) 127
  Thiamine (Vitamin B1) 128

Part VIII
Respiratory & Pulmonary Meds 129
  Albuterol (Proventil, Ventolin) 131
  Ipratropium (Atrovent) 132
  Succinylcholine (Anectine) 133
  Terbutaline (Brethine) 134

Part IX
Antipsychotics, Antiemetics & Miscellaneous 135
  Droperidol (Inapsine) 137
  Glycopyrrolate (Robinul) 138
  Haloperidol (Haldol) 139
  Olanzapine (Zyprexa) 140
  Ondansetron (Zofran) 141
  Prochlorperazine (Compazine) 142
  Promethazine (Phenergan) 143
  Ziprasidone (Geodon) 144

Part X
Neuromuscular Blockers & Reversal 145
  Cisatracurium (Nimbex) 147
  Rocuronium (Zemuron) 148
  Sugammadex 149
  Vecuronium (Norcuron) 150

Part XI
Fluids, Electrolytes, and ICU-Specific 151
  Calcium Chloride 153
  Calcium Gluconate 154
  Furosemide (Lasix) 155
  Hydrocortisone (Solu-Cortef) 156
  Hypertonic Saline (3% Sodium Chloride) 157
  Hypertonic Saline (7.5%) 158
  Hypertonic Saline (23.4%) 159
  Labetalol (Trandate, Normodyne) 160
  Magnesium Sulfate 161
  Mannitol (Bronchitol) 162
  Methylprednisolone (Solu-Medrol) 163
  Tetanus Immune Globulin (TIG) 164

WHY Made Easy Works

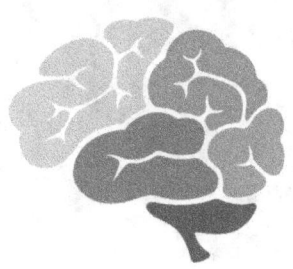

Backed by Brain Science

Let's face it — nursing school can feel like trying to drink from a firehose. Between the jargon, the never-ending lists, and the sheer volume of information, it's easy to feel overwhelmed. That's exactly why the Made Easy series was born: to make the hard stuff stick without frying your brain. And while it might look fun and playful on the outside (hello, rhymes!), it's all built on rock-solid research from the nerdy world of educational psychology.

1. COGNITIVE LOAD THEORY

First up: Cognitive Load Theory. Fancy name, simple idea — your brain can only handle so much at once. When materials are too dense or packed with fluff, your working memory taps out. Educational psychologist John Sweller figured this out, and we took notes. That's why our poems give you the essentials only, in small, memorable doses. Less clutter, more clarity. (Sweller, 1988; Clark et al., 2006)

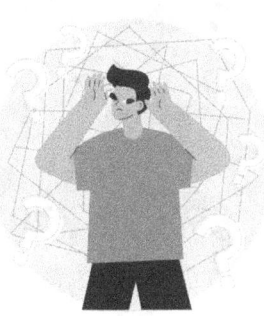

2. DUAL CODING THEORY

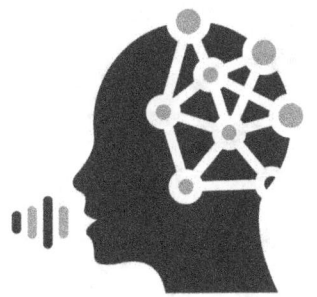

Then there's Dual Coding Theory, brought to us by Allan Paivio. He discovered that we remember things better when we learn them through both words and visuals. Our poems lean into this by using rhyme and rhythm to boost verbal memory — and bolded key terms, color coding, and clean formatting to give your visual brain a treat. Two paths to your brain = double the retention. (Paivio, 1986; Mayer, 2009)

3. ADVANCE ORGANIZERS

Psychologist David Ausubel believed that when we know how new info fits into what we already know, we learn faster. That's the beauty of our repeatable poem structure. Once you get the hang of the format, your brain relaxes — and focuses on what actually matters: the content. Think of it like a familiar playlist for your mind. (Ausubel, 1960)

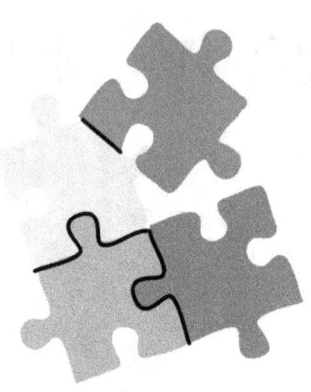

4. MICROLEARNING

Our poems are also bite-sized by design, and that's no accident. Welcome to the world of microlearning — the idea that small, focused learning units are easier to digest and retain. This is a game-changer for busy, burnt-out students. Instead of cramming for hours, you can study just one medication, one skill, or one critical concept at a time. Snack-sized studying with full-course impact. (Hug, 2005; van den Berg & van den Berg, 2021)

5. SPACED REPETITION & RETRIEVAL PRACTICE

Last but definitely not least: spaced repetition and retrieval practice. These two learning powerhouses have proven time and again that the more often you recall information over time, the longer you'll remember it. Our poems are made for this. Easy to reread, perfect for flashcards, and fun enough to come back to (yes, we admitted it). Rinse and repeat — and retain. (Dunlosky et al., 2013)

So, yes — this method might look different than your typical textbook grind. That's the point. It's effective on purpose. Because learning tough topics shouldn't feel impossible. It should feel doable. Even a little fun. And with Made Easy, it totally is.

Read it. Rhyme it. Remember it.

That's the Made Easy Method—a simple but powerful approach to mastering complex nursing material.

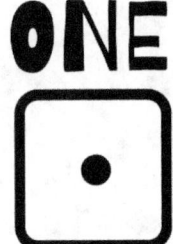

START WITH THE BIG PICTURE

Before diving into individual medications, review the Mind Maps (via QR code). These quick-reference visuals give you the foundational understanding needed for any medication.

Included mind maps:
- The Life of a Drug in the Body (pharmacokinetics)
- Drug Classifications
- Common Side Effect Categories
- High-Risk Medication Categories
- Drug Schedules (I-V)
- Therapeutic Index & Drug Monitoring
- Common Drug Interactions
- Ways to Memorize Meds

These are perfect for test prep, concept review, and connecting the dots across drug types.

USE THE MEMORY TRICKS & MNEMONICS

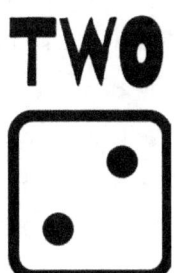

We've included 2 pages of mnemonic "cards" – visual reminders of popular phrases and acronyms students actually use (and remember!).

Cut them out, hang them up, or snap a pic to review on the go.

THREE

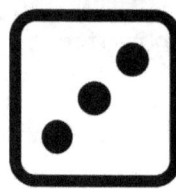

STUDY WITH PURPOSE

Don't just read — actively study.
As you go through each medication, we encourage you to highlight or underline using this color-coded system to instantly recognize what's what:

- ▪ Drug Classification & Names
- ▪ Mechanism of Action
- ▪ Indications
- ▪ Side Effects & Adverse Reactions
- ▪ Nursing Considerations
- ▪ Monitoring Requirements
- ▪ Patient & Caregiver Teaching Points
- ● Black Box Warnings
- ▪ Pediatric Considerations
- ● Drug Interactions

(Pro Tip: You don't need 10 highlighters — just make a little color key and underline or box with gel pens or colored pencils!)

COMPLETE THE MIND MAP

FOUR

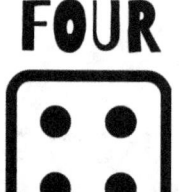

Once you've highlighted, it's time to organize what you've learned. Use the Medication Mind Map Template in the back of the book to visually break down the drug:

- Class, MOA, Indications
- Side effects, warnings, teaching points
- Your favorite memory trick or mnemonic

This helps you actually process and remember what you just studied — way better than passive reading.

FIVE
TEST WHAT YOU KNOW

After each section, you'll find a QR code that takes you straight to a short NCLEX-style quiz hosted in Google Forms. These aren't just random practice questions — they're carefully crafted to test the most important takeaways from what you just read. But the real magic? <u>The rationales.</u> Whether you get the answer right or wrong, the quiz walks you through the why. Understanding the reasoning behind each answer helps you think like a nurse, not just a test-taker.

It's not about memorizing — it's about making connections, strengthening critical thinking, and applying your knowledge in real clinical scenarios. So take your time, review the rationales, and let them guide you from confusion to clarity.

So don't just read these pages—
interact with them.

📖 Read it. 🎵 Rhyme it. 🧠 Remember it.

> Nursing is an art: and if it is to be made an art, it requires an exclusive devotion as hard a preparation as any painter's or sculptor's work.
> - Florence Nightingale

PHARMACOLOGY MIND MAPS

COMMON DRUG INTERACTIONS

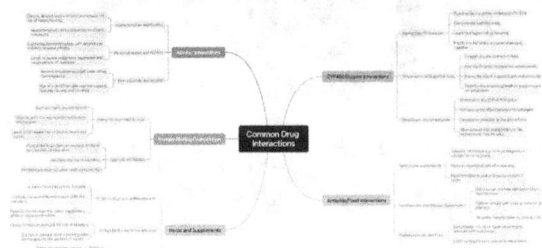

THE LIFE OF A DRUG IN THE BODY

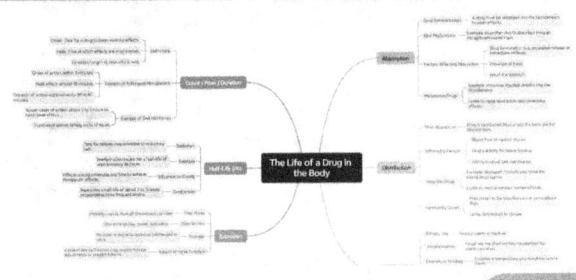

DRUG CLASSIFICATIONS

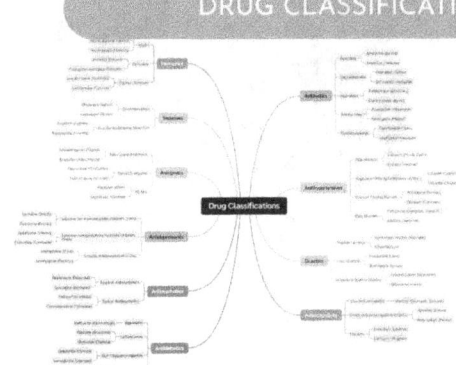

HIGH-RISK MEDICATION CATEGORIES

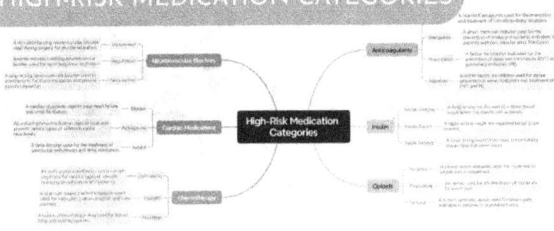

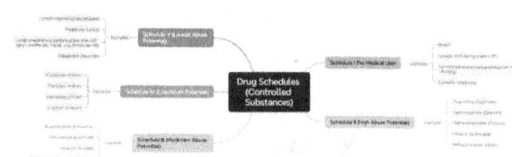

DRUG SCHEDULES

THERAPEUTIC INDEX & DRUG MONITORING

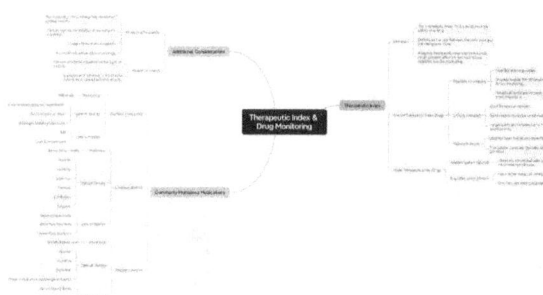

COMMON DRUG INTERACTIONS

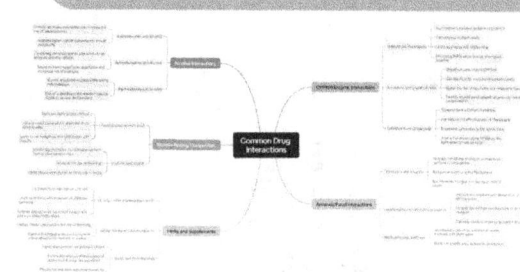

WAYS TO MEMORIZE MEDICATIONS

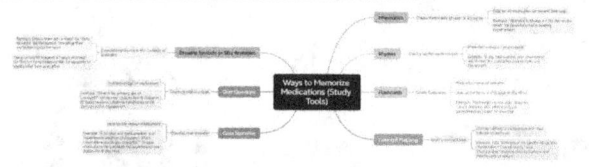

Pharm Mnemonics

SLUDGE
CHOLINERGIC EFFECTS

Salivation, **L**acrimation, **U**rination, **D**iaphoresis, **G**I upset, **E**mesis

Seen in cholinergic overdose or organophosphate poisoning.

ANTICHOLINERGIC
Can't Pee, See, Spit, or Poop

Blurred vision, Urinary retention, Dry mouth, Constipation

Helps recall the hallmark side effects of anticholinergic medications.

NAMES OF INSULINS - L.A.N.D.

Lantus = Long-acting
Apidra = Rapid-acting
Novolog = Rapid-acting
Detemir = Long-acting

BETA-BLOCKERS

"**LOL** Makes the Heart Rate Slow"

All beta-blockers end in "-lol." They decrease heart rate and blood pressure by blocking beta-adrenergic receptors.

ACE INHIBITORS

"**-PRIL** Puts the Pressure Down"

Pressure Reduced In Large vessels. They lower blood pressure by preventing angiotensin II formation.

CALCIUM CHANNEL BLOCKERS

"**V**ery **N**ice **D**rugs"
Verapamil, **N**ifedipine, **D**iltiazem

These drugs dilate blood vessels and slow the heart rate, reducing workload on the heart.

DIURETICS

"**DIM** the Fluid Volume"

Diuretics, **I**ncrease, **M**icturition (urination)

Loop diuretics (e.g., furosemide) or thiazides (e.g., hydrochlorothiazide) help reduce fluid volume, easing edema or hypertension.

ANTICOAGULANTS

"Heparin Works **FAST**, Coumadin **LASTS**"

Heparin is for acute management; Warfarin for long-term prevention. Always monitor lab values (PTT for heparin, PT/INR for warfarin).

ANTIBIOTICS (PENICILLINS & CEPHALOSPORINS)

"Cross Allergy Alerts"

All beta-blockers end in "-lol." They decrease heart rate and blood pressure by blocking beta-adrenergic receptors.

LIDOCAINE TOXICITY

"**SAMS**"
Slurred speech, **A**ltered central nervous system, **M**uscle twitching, **S**eizures

Recognize signs of lidocaine toxicity.

MEDICATION ADMINISTRATION CHECKLIST

"**TRAMP**"

Time, **R**oute, **A**mount, **M**edication, **P**atient

Ensure the five rights of medication administration.

EMERGENCY DRUGS TO "**LEAN**" ON

Lidocaine, **E**pinephrine, **A**tropine, **N**aloxone

Common emergency medications administered via endotracheal tube.

Pharm Mnemonics

VENTRICULAR ARRHYTHMIAS
"PALS"
Procainamide, **A**miodarone, **L**idocaine, **S**otalol

Medications used to treat ventricular arrhythmias.

ATRIAL ARRHYTHMIAS
"ABCDE"
Anticoagulants, **B**eta blockers, **C**alcium channel blockers, **D**igoxin, **E**lectrocardioversion

Treatment options for atrial arrhythmias.

MORPHINE SIDE EFFECTS
"MORPHINE"
Miosis, **O**ut of it (sedation), **R**espiratory depression, **P**neumonia (aspiration), **H**ypotension, **I**nfrequency (constipation, urinary retention), **N**ausea, **E**mesis

PARKINSON'S MEDICATIONS
"ALBM"
Amantadine, **L**evodopa, **B**romocriptine, **M**AO-B inhibitors

Drugs commonly used to manage Parkinson's disease.

THIAZIDES INDICATIONS
"CHIC"
Congestive heart failure, **H**ypertension, **I**nsipidus (diabetes insipidus), **C**alcium calculi (kidney stones)

Primary uses for thiazide diuretics.

BRADYCARDIA & HYPOTENSION
"IDEA"
Isoproterenol, **D**opamine, **E**pinephrine, **A**tropine sulfate

Medications used to manage bradycardia and hypotension.

STEROID SIDE EFFECTS
"6 S's"
Sugar - hyperglycemia, **S**oggy bones - osteoporosis, **S**ick - decreased immunity, **S**ad - depression, **S**alt - water and salt retention, **S**ex - decreased libido

LOOP DIURETIC EFFECTS
"LOOP"
Lose sodium, **O**totoxicity, **O**rthostatic hypotension, **P**otassium loss

Highlights the primary effects and risks of loop diuretics.

ACE INHIBITOR SIDE EFFECTS
"CAPTOPRIL"
Cough, **A**ngioedema, **P**roteinuria, **T**aste changes, **O**rthostatic hypotension, **P**regnancy contraindication, **R**ash, **I**ncreased renin, **L**ower angiotensin II

BETA-BLOCKER CONTRAINDICATIONS
"ABCDE"
Asthma, **B**lock (heart block), **C**OPD, **D**iabetes mellitus, **E**lectrolyte (hyperkalemia)

Highlights conditions where beta-blockers should be used cautiously or avoided.

GYNECOMASTIA
"DISCO"
Digitalis, **I**soniazid, **S**pironolactone, **C**imetidine, **O**estrogens

Identifies medications known to cause gynecomastia as a side effect.

TOXICOLOGICAL SEIZURES
"OTIS CAMPBELL"
Organophosphates, **T**ricyclic antidepressants, **I**soniazid, **I**nsulin, **S**ympathomimetics, **C**amphor, **C**ocaine, **A**mphetamines, **M**ethylxanthines, **P**CP, **P**ropoxyphene, **P**henol, **P**ropranolol, **B**enzodiazepine withdrawal, **B**otanicals, **E**thanol withdrawal, **L**ithium, **L**idocaine, **L**indane, **L**ead

Part I
Analgesics, Antipyretics & Sedation

ACETAMINOPHEN (TYLENOL)

Non-opioid Analgesic / Antipyretic

A common name that's widely known,
Acetaminophen stands alone.
A **non-opioid** for pain relief,
And **fevers** too, it brings you peace.
It blocks the brain's **COX enzyme path**,
But skips inflammation's wrath.
So **analgesia** it imparts,
And **fever reduction** plays a part.

Mild to moderate pain it treats,
For **headaches**, strains, or aching feet.
Also lowers fevers high—
A **go-to med**, and here is why:
It's **generally safe**, but don't go wild,
Too much can make the **liver riled**.
Hepatotoxicity is the scare,
Especially when you're unaware.

Watch for **nausea, sweating,** chills,
Or upper pain that lingers still.
A **rash or hives** may sometimes show—
Then **stop the med** and let them know.
Nurses: check the56qq **dose** they take,
And all the meds for overlap's sake.
Because it hides in combo blends—
Read those labels to the end.

Keep tabs on **liver function labs**,
Especially when the dose is drab.
ALT, AST, and **bilirubin** too,
To spot the damage coming through.
Teach the patient: don't exceed
4 grams per day, that is the need.
Warn them drinking **alcohol**
Could make the liver take a fall.

Black box warning: though not yet stamped,
Overdose is where things get cramped.
It's one of the top calls made—
For **toxicity**, seek NAC aid.
Beware of drugs that also work
On **CYP enzymes**, or they may lurk
To **raise the risk** of liver strain—
Like **phenytoin**, or **warfarin**'s gain.

So use with care and check each dose,
This med is simple, yet quite close
To causing harm if not reviewed—
Acetaminophen, rightly used.

DEXAMETHASONE (DECADRON)
Corticosteroid - Glucocorticoid

Dexamethasone brings down the flame,
Inflammation is its game.
A **steroid** strong with lasting might,
It calms the body's inner fight.
Used in **cancer, asthma, brain edema**,
Allergic reactions, and **COVID** schema.
Also helps in **shock, nausea**, too—
And **autoimmune** when flares break through.

It mimics **cortisol** from glands,
With far-reaching **anti-inflammatory** hands.
But it comes with a lengthy list—
Of **side effects** nurses can't miss.
Hyperglycemia, mood swings, weight gain,
Cushing's syndrome may explain.
GI bleeding, insomnia, bone loss slow,
And **immune suppression** head to toe.

Can raise **BP**, and drop **K+**,
So monitor **labs**—don't ever guess.
Check **blood sugar, weight**, and mood,
And **signs of infection**, though they're subdued.
Teach to **never stop abruptly**, friend—
Or **adrenal crisis** may descend.
Taper slowly, doctor's plan,
Or **hypotension** hits the fan.

Take with **food** to guard the belly,
And report if stools turn **black and jelly**.
Also warn of **facial swelling**,
Or **vision changes** that need telling.
No **Black Box Warning**, but long-term stay
Means side effects may find their way.
It **interacts** with **NSAIDs, vaccines**, and more—
So review meds before you pour.

Dexamethasone, a mighty friend,
But nursing care must never bend.
With **labs, teaching**, and **daily check**,
You'll keep this steroid safe on deck.

DIAZEPAM (VALIUM)

Benzodiazepine – Anxiolytic, Anticonvulsant, Muscle Relaxant

Diazepam, a calming breeze,
Brings **anxiety** and **seizures** to ease.
A **benzodiazepine**, tried and true,
It **boosts GABA**—the brain's brake crew.
Used in **anxiety, seizure control**,
And **muscle spasms** that take a toll.
Also helps with **alcohol withdrawal**,
And **sedation** needs before it all.
It works to **slow the CNS down**,
Relieves the jitters, chills, and frown.
But don't forget the sleepy side—
Drowsiness, fatigue, and **falls worldwide**.
Respiratory depression is the scare,
Especially when **IV** or **mixed with care**.
So monitor **rate and depth of breath**,
And guard against **sedation death**.
Watch for signs of **dependence** deep—
It's not a drug for lifelong keep.
Withdrawal seizures can occur
If stopped too fast—it may deter.
Flumazenil is the **antidote**,
If **overdose** makes breathing bloat.
But use with caution, don't forget—
It may bring **seizure risk** or threat.
Black Box Warning—you must know:
Combined with **opioids**, risk will grow.
The mix may cause **coma, death**, or more,
So nurse, be cautious at the core.
It interacts with drugs galore—
Like **alcohol, CNS depressants**, and more.
Also **cimetidine, valproate**,
May boost the levels at a rate.
Teach patients not to **drive or drink**,
Until they know how slow they think.
Warn about **tolerance** setting in,
And **withdrawal symptoms** creeping in.
Diazepam—relief with rules,
For **seizures, spasms**, and anxious duels.
With skillful hands and patient trust,
You'll use this benzo right and just.

7

DEXMEDETOMIDINE (PRECEDEX)
Sedative - Alpha-2 Adrenergic Agonist

Dexmedetomidine, smooth and wise,
Sedates the brain, but keeps the eyes.
It **activates alpha-2** in the brain,
To slow down **norepinephrine's train**.
Used for **sedation without full knock-out**,
In **ICUs** and **surgical routes**.
Keeps patients calm, but **arousable**,
And breathing on their own—quite valuable!

Helps in **intubation**, light **anesthesia**,
Or **weaning off vents** without amnesia.
It eases **anxiety**, pain, and fear,
Without the crash some meds bring near.
Side effects may still arise:
Bradycardia, **hypotension**, compromise.
Also **dry mouth**, and sometimes chills,
As sedation gently fills.

Monitor **BP**, and **heart rate**, too,
It **drops the pulse**—sometimes like glue.
Don't give **rapid IV push**,
It can cause a **hemodynamic crush**.

No **Black Box Warning**, but nurse take note:
Watch vitals **closely**, keep afloat.
It's **not for long-term sedation** plans,
Use with care per ICU scans.

Avoid use with **other CNS depressants**,
Or **opioids**—may increase side effects present.
Also caution in **heart block states**,
Or if **severe liver** complicates.
Teach the team: Though patient sleeps,
They still may hear and **feel things deep**.
Always assess for **pain and needs**,
And document sedation speeds.

Dexmedetomidine—calm and clear,
A mindful sedative when you're near.
For nurses trained and watching right,
It helps the stormy shift feel light.

DIPHENHYDRAMINE (BENADRYL)

Antihistamine – First-Generation H1 Blocker

Diphenhydramine, old but strong,
Blocks histamine when things go wrong.
An **H1 blocker**, first in line,
To stop the **itch**, the **rash**, the **sneeze** in time.
Used for **allergies**, **hives**, **runny nose**,
Insomnia, and **motion woes**.
Also helps with **anaphylaxis**,
Though **epinephrine** leads that axis.

It causes **CNS sedation** quick,
So don't let grandma take it slick.
Think **drowsiness**, **dizziness**, **dry mouth**, too,
And **urinary retention** out of the blue.
It's got **anticholinergic traits**,
So **can't see, can't pee** kind of states.
Constipation, **dry eyes**, and more,
Especially when the dose does soar.

Elderly caution is a must—
Falls and **confusion** breach their trust.
May worsen **dementia** and **cognitive fog**,
Or make them sleep like a log.
No Black Box Warning, but still beware—
It's **not for infants** or **young child care**.
Watch for **paradoxical effects**,
Like **hyperactivity** in some contexts.

It **interacts** with **alcohol**, **opioids**, too,
And other meds that **slow the crew**.
Also **MAOIs** can raise the risk,
Of **CNS depression** that's brisk.
Teach patients: **Don't drive** or drink a drop,
Until you know if the **drowsy will stop**.
And don't **combine** with sleep meds stacked—
Too much chill, and breath gets cracked.

Diphenhydramine—helpful and cheap,
But use it safe, or it cuts too deep.
For **itch and sneeze** or **nights without sleep**,
This med is strong, not just skin-deep.

ETOMIDATE (AMIDATE)

General Anesthetic – Sedative-Hypnotic
(Non-Barbiturate)

Etomidate, quick and clean,
A **sedative-hypnotic** in the scene.
Used for **rapid sequence intubation**,
It brings a calm, near **insta-sedation**.
It works on the **GABA receptors** tight,
To dim the brain and shut the light.
It does **not relieve pain**, so plan ahead—
Pair with **opioids** if pain is spread.

Given **IV**, it acts real fast,
But wears off quick—it doesn't last.
Perfect for **short-term procedural sleep**,
Or when airway control is what you keep.
Side effects you need to watch:
Myoclonus, nausea, even **hormone botch**.
It can **suppress adrenal glands**,
So check for **cortisol crash** in plans.

Hypotension is rare but real,
Especially in those who're already ill.
Respiratory depression? Not much seen—
That's why it's loved in the **trauma scene**.

No Black Box Warning, but stay aware,
It's **not for long-term sedation care**.
And if your patient has **sepsis stress**,
Its **adrenal block** may cause a mess.

Monitor vitals every beat,
Keep the airway clear and neat.
Have **crash cart ready**, suction, too,
Even though it's stable through and through.
Teach your team: **Pain control** is still due,
This med just makes the mind go mute.
So **pre-medicate or follow through**
With **analgesia**, not just a snooze.

Etomidate—a calm and quick dive,
For **airway care** or **sedation to thrive**.
In skilled nurse hands, it earns its name,
Keeping patients safe in the intubation game.

FENTANYL (SUBLIMAZE)
Opioid Analgesic - Schedule II Controlled Substance

Fentanyl, a **pain reliever** strong,
A **synthetic opioid** that doesn't take long.
100 times stronger than morphine's dose,
So **tiny amounts** mean serious close.
Used for **surgical pain**, **sedation**, too,
In **patch**, **IV**, or **buccal** view.
Also for **chronic pain control**,
In patients who are opioid-pro.

It binds to **mu receptors** fast,
To stop the pain and make it pass.
But nurses, know the risks it brings—
This med can **depress respiratory things**.
Side effects to monitor near:
Respiratory depression, the biggest fear.
Also **bradycardia**, **constipation**,
Sedation, **nausea**, and **confusion station**.

It's **short-acting IV**, so in a flash,
It helps in trauma or surgical crash.
But **patches** last for days, be warned—
So **rotate sites** and **heat avoid**—they're scorned.
Black Box Warning? Yes, it's true:
Respiratory arrest can ensue.
Especially when **mixed with CNS depressants**,
Or used by those without opioid lessons.

Naloxone is the **antidote**,
Have it ready—don't just hope.
Monitor **RR**, **O₂ sat**, too,
And assess the **pain scale through and through**.
Teach patients: **No alcohol** or sleep meds stacked,
This combo could cause lungs to slack.
Watch for **drowsiness** or delayed speech,
And **call for help** if breath seems out of reach.

Fentanyl—potent, fast, and bold,
But best when nurse's hands take hold.
With teaching, care, and eyes alert,
You'll ease the pain without the hurt.

HYDROMORPHONE (DILAUDID)

Hydromorphone, strong and tight,
A **pain reliever** with serious bite.
It binds to **mu receptors** in the brain,
To block **pain signals**, dull the strain.
It's **7 times stronger** than morphine's way,
So dose it low and monitor all day.
Used in **severe pain, trauma, cancer**,
It works real fast—but needs a dancer.

Side effects? They're not small:
Respiratory depression most of all.
Also **sedation, nausea**, and **itch**,
Constipation is in the pitch.
Watch for **hypotension, bradycardia**, too,
Especially when **IV dosing** is due.
And if you see **cyanosis, snore**,
Check that **O₂ sat** and **respiratory score**.

Black Box Warning sits on this med:
For **addiction, abuse**, and **death** widespread.
Especially with **benzos** or **alcohol**,
The **CNS depression** can make them fall.

Naloxone (Narcan) is the key,
The **antidote** for breathing free.
Have it close if dosing high,
To guard the breath and not the sigh.

Give **slow IV**—don't ever push,
Fast dosing can cause **hypotensive rush**.
And if **oral**, give with care,
Explain the risks and side effects there.
Teach: **No driving, no wine, no weed**,
Until they know how they'll proceed.
And **increase fluids, fiber, stool softener aid**,
To keep that opioid gut parade.

Hydromorphone—potent, pure,
But only safe with nurse's cure.
With eyes on **rate**, and skills on deck,
You'll guide this med with perfect check.

IBUPROFEN (ADVIL, MOTRIN)

NSAID – Nonsteroidal Anti-Inflammatory Drug

Ibuprofen, pain's quick end,
A common over-the-counter friend.
It **blocks COX-1 and COX-2** tight,
To **stop prostaglandins** in their fight.
Used for **pain, fever, inflammation**,
Arthritis, cramps, or **menstruation**.
Also helpful in **muscle strain**,
But take with caution to avoid **pain's gain**.

Side effects may come in packs:
GI upset, and **heartburn attacks**.
Long-term use may cause **ulcers** deep,
So teach your patients not to leap.
GI bleeding, **black stools**, red throw-up,
Should stop this drug and get a check-up.
And **kidney damage** is a fear—
So monitor **BUN and creatinine** near.

Raises BP, can **worsen heart**,
So avoid in patients with **cardiac start**.
And in **asthma**, use with care,
It may provoke a wheezy scare.
Black Box Warnings—yes, two clear:
For **GI bleeds** and **heart attacks** near.

Not for **CABG surgery pain**,
As risk of **clot** and **death** is plain.

Interacts with many meds in kind,
Like **ACE inhibitors**, which you'll find
Can worsen **renal function** when paired,
So watch the labs and be prepared.
Teach to take it **with some food**,
And not to mix in reckless mood.
No alcohol, and don't stack high,
Keep dose below **3200 mg** per try.

Ibuprofen—cheap and quick,
But risks can make the patient sick.
With teaching, checks, and nursing might,
You'll use this med just right and tight.

KETAMINE (KETALAR)
Dissociative Anesthetic

Induction and **sedation**, it's often portrayed,
Used in the OR, in trauma, with aid.
Rapid-acting IV—a dissociative trance,
Brings on a fog and a faraway glance.
It blocks the **NMDA receptor's control**,
Reducing **pain signals** from reaching the soul.
You get **amnesia**, **analgesia**, too—
While breathing stays stable (a helpful breakthrough).

Used for **intubation** or **RSI**,
Or **depression resistant**—it's gaining some sky.
Low-dose infusions for chronic pain care,
A **non-opioid** option when others aren't there.
Watch for **hallucinations**, they're vivid and loud,
Or **increased ICP**—not safe for that crowd.
It causes **tachycardia**, **pressure may rise**,
But breathing's preserved—that's quite a prize.

Avoid in **glaucoma** or **brain trauma past**,
If **ICP's high**, it could backfire fast.
Be cautious with **psychosis**, it may amplify,
The mind dissociates, lets the body lie.
Administer gently, reduce too much light,
A **benzo** may help ease the journey at night.
Monitor vitals, keep suction nearby,
Prepare for a trip—don't let safety slide by.

So **Ketamine**, potent, dissociative, fast—
A unique anesthetic, with effects that last.
Used wisely, it helps both the body and brain,
In surgeries deep or to soften deep pain.

KETOROLAC (TORADOL)
NSAID (Nonsteroidal Anti-Inflammatory Drug)

It's **not a narcotic**, but pain it can tame,
Ketorolac's power earns it strong name.
For **moderate pain**, it works super well,
Especially IV, it starts to excel.
It blocks the **COX enzymes**, both **one and two**,
To reduce **prostaglandins** and inflammation too.
You'll see less **swelling**, less **fever**, less **ache**,
But protect the **GI**, for ulcer's sake.

It's often used **post-op** or **acute ER pain**,
But only for **5 days**, or side effects reign.
GI bleeding and **renal decline**
Are reasons this drug has a tight line.
Avoid in **bleeding**, or **peptic ulcer disease**,
And **renal impairment**—it won't please.
Don't mix with **other NSAIDs**—the risks combine,
And be cautious in **elderly**, every time.

No use in **labor**, it might close the duct,
The **ductus arteriosus**—a fetal construct.
It can cause **hypertension**, or impact the plate,
So check labs and vitals—don't underestimate.

It's **not addictive**, and doesn't sedate,
But it's powerful—used to alternate.
Rotate with **opioids** or use alone,
But monitor closely once it's shown.

So **Toradol's** strong, but time-limited gear,
A **non-opioid** warrior nurses revere.
Short term relief—used smart, not bold,
And always with **risks** clearly told.

LIDOCAINE (XYLOCAINE)
Local Anesthetic & Antiarrhythmic (Class 1B)

For **numbing the skin** or calming the heart,
Lidocaine plays a versatile part.
Injected for pain or applied to a patch,
It **blocks sodium channels**, a fast-acting catch.
In **local anesthesia**, it dulls the feel,
Before a **procedure**, or closing a seal.
In dental, dermal, and minor repair,
It numbs the nerves with precision and care.

But it's also used when **arrhythmias rise**,
Like **ventricular tachy** or deadly **V-fib surprise**.
Given **IV** in emergent care,
It slows the heart's rhythm with expert flair.
Side effects can come if the dose gets high—
CNS toxicity can amplify.
Watch for **tremors**, **seizures**, **confusion**, or **slur**,
Or **hypotension**, and rhythm that's a blur.

Avoid in those with **heart blocks** or brady,
And **hepatic impairment**—check labs already.
Caution with **elderly**, and give at the rate

That's **slow and steady**, to lower the fate.
Topically used, it's quite well-behaved,
But don't use on **open wounds** or **shaved**.
Watch for **systemic absorption** risk,
Especially with **large areas**—not worth the frisk.

So **Lidocaine**, flexible, fast, and slick,
For **pain** or **arrhythmias**, it does the trick.
But dosing must be sharp and wise,
To keep this drug a helpful prize.

LORAZEPAM (ATIVAN)
Benzodiazepine (Anxiolytic, Sedative, Anticonvulsant)

Lorazepam's calming—it chills the brain,
It boosts **GABA** so nerves feel less strain.
Used for **anxiety**, **panic**, and more,
And **seizures**, even **status** you can't ignore.
It's helpful before **surgery**, keeps people still,
Or to ease **withdrawal** when **alcohol's ill**.
It **relaxes muscles**, helps **insomnia**, too,
A benzo with many things it can do.

But side effects come—**sedation**, **slurred speech**,
Drowsy, **dizzy**, with a long reach.
It depresses the **CNS**, so take care,
Especially mixed with **opioids**—a dangerous pair.
It may cause **dependence**, so short term is best,
Watch for **withdrawal** if stopping the rest.
Taper it slowly, don't stop in a snap,
Or rebound symptoms could set a trap.

Given **IV**, it works real fast,
In **seizures**, that's helpful—it acts so vast.
But monitor closely: **RR and BP**,
And **LOC**—how alert they be.
Avoid alcohol, and don't drive around,
Until you know how the drug's going down.

In **older adults**, use lower dose,
It can cause **falls** or **delirium** the most.

So **Lorazepam**, soothing but strong,
Used carefully, it won't steer you wrong.
For **panic, seizures**, or surgical prep,
This med earns respect with every step.

MIDAZOLAM (VERSED)
Benzodiazepine - Sedative/Hypnotic, Anxiolytic

Midazolam, smooth and fast,
A **benzo** that doesn't last.
It brings on **calm**, **sedation deep**,
Before a scope or surgical sleep.
Used for **procedural sedation** needs,
Or **pre-op anxiety** that speeds.
Also helps in **status epilepticus**,
When seizures try to take control of us.
It binds to **GABA receptors tight**,
To enhance the brain's **inhibitory light**.
Given **IV**, **IM**, or **intranasal**,
Its onset is nearly **sensational**.
Side effects to watch with care:
Respiratory depression is always there.
Also **bradycardia, hypotension** low,
And **drowsiness** that takes it slow.
It can cause **amnesia**—they won't recall,
Which may be good in a procedure hall.
But also leads to **confusion, fear**,
When waking up feels unclear.
Black Box Warning shouts aloud:
Respiratory arrest can form a cloud—
Especially when mixed with **opioids** tight,
So monitor breathing **day and night**.
Keep **resuscitation** tools at side,
And **flumazenil** nearby to guide.

That's the **antidote** if things go wrong,
But use it slow—it doesn't last long.
Monitor vitals every bit,
And stay bedside—**never quit**.
This drug is **high alert** in hand,
So **double-check** before you stand.
Teach the patient: **No alcohol**,
And **no driving** till you make the call.
They might forget the whole next day,
So keep instructions clear and stay.

Midazolam—a peaceful ride,
But only safe with nurse beside.
With skills, eyes sharp, and airway prepped,
You'll use this benzo with respect.

MORPHINE

Opioid Analgesic - Schedule II Controlled Substance

Morphine, classic, strong, and deep,
Relieves the pain, helps patients sleep.
It binds to **mu receptors** fast,
To make the pain and struggle pass.
Used for **moderate to severe pain**,
MI, **trauma**, or **post-op strain**.
Also helps in **pulmonary edema**,
By easing **anxiety** and **breathing schema**.
Given **oral**, **IV**, **IM**, or **subQ**,
Even **rectal** or **epidural** too.
But dose with care and watch the signs—
This med can **cross many lines**.
Side effects to check and chart:
Respiratory depression is the start.
Constipation, hypotension, sedation,
Nausea, vomiting, and **urine retention**.
Can cause **itching**, **euphoria** high,
Or **dependence** if it's long supplied.
Tolerance, addiction, and **abuse**
Are risks with every opioid use.
Black Box Warning stands its ground:
Respiratory arrest can come around.
Especially when mixed with **benzos**, booze,
Or given fast without good cues.
Naloxone (Narcan) is your friend,
To **reverse the opiate** at the end.
Have it nearby when doses climb,
And monitor **RR** every time.
Check **pain level** before and after,
And reassess their breath and chatter.

Avoid **alcohol**, and don't combine
With other **CNS depressants** in line.
Teach: Take it **exactly as prescribed**,
And keep it safe, where kids won't dive.
Stool softeners often come along,
Because **opioid gut** is stubborn strong.

Morphine—potent, classic, pure,
But only safe when checks are sure.
With nursing skill and patient trust,
You'll use this med the way you must.

OXYCODONE (OXYCONTIN, ROXICODONE)

Opioid Analgesic - Schedule II Controlled Substance

Oxycodone, pain's retreat,
For aches that run incredibly deep.
It binds to **mu receptors** tight,
To block the pain and calm the fight.
Used for **moderate to severe pain**,
In **post-op**, **injury**, or **chronic strain**.
It comes in forms both **IR** and **ER**,
But always monitor from near.
Immediate release (Roxicodone) starts fast,
While **OxyContin** makes the relief last.
But both can cause that classic ride—
Euphoria, sleepiness, pain denied.
Side effects you must report:
Respiratory depression—nurse's court.
Also **sedation, nausea, itch**,
And **constipation** that doesn't switch.
Black Box Warning calls aloud:
Addiction, abuse, and **death** are vowed.
Especially when **combined with benzos**, booze—
It's **CNS depression** you can't afford to lose.
Tolerance and **dependence** can grow,
So assess the patient **before you go**.
Check **pain scale, RR, BP, LOC**,
And **hold the dose** if breathing's low.

Naloxone (Narcan) is your plan,
If overdose grabs the upper hand.
Have it nearby, and teach it, too—
For home use when scripts go through.
Teach: No driving or drinking wine,
Take the med **on schedule, not on a whim line**.
And use a **stool softener** right from the start,
To keep things moving and do their part.
Don't crush extended-release, please,
It can cause a fatal release.
Swallow whole and store away—
Out of reach where kids don't play.
Oxycodone—relief in strain,
But not without its risks and pain.
With nurse-led checks and honest talk,
You'll guide this med like a steady rock.

PROPOFOL (DIPRIVAN)
General Anesthetic - Sedative-Hypnotic (IV Only)

Propofol, milky, smooth, and fast,
Brings on **sedation** that doesn't last.
A **GABA-activator**, deep and wide,
That puts the **CNS** to sleep inside.
Used for **intubation, surgery, sedation care**,
In the **ICU** or the **OR** chair.
Also helps in **vented** patients rest,
So the body can heal and feel less stressed.

IV only, don't give by mouth,
And always **infuse**—never bolus south.
Onset? Seconds. Wears off quick,
But needs a nurse who's sharp and slick.
Side effects include these signs:
Bradycardia, hypotensive lines.
And **respiratory depression** strong—
So **airway gear** won't steer you wrong.

Watch for rare but serious tale:
Propofol Infusion Syndrome—can derail.
Seen in **long-term, high-dose** infusion,
With **metabolic acidosis**, cardiac confusion.
Can raise **lipids**, cause **green urine**,
Odd, but safe—so don't start stewin'.
But this med feeds **bacteria quick**,
So **change tubing every 12** like a pro pick.

Monitor **RR, BP**, and state of mind,
Though memory loss is by design.
Not a **controlled substance** by the book,
But still gets **abused**—so take a look.
No Black Box Warning, but still with might,
This med demands **nurse oversight**.
With careful pumps and steady grace,
You'll keep this drip in the safest place.

Propofol—a sedative strong,
But safe in skilled hands all shift long.
With nurse precision, and keen bedside,
You'll guide this med with calm and pride.

Part II
Cardiovascular & Hemodynamic Support

ADENOSINE (ADENOCARD)
Antiarrhythmic - Class V

Adenosine, a cardiac friend,
Used when rhythms twist or bend.
A **Class V antiarrhythmic drug**,
It gives the heart a needed tug.
It **slows conduction through the AV node**,
A brief **heart pause** is often showed.
Interrupts reentry pathways fast,
So **PSVT** won't long last.
Indications? Here they go:
Paroxysmal supraventricular tachycardia (PSVT) to slow.
Also used in **stress tests** too—
To mimic work the heart might do.
But side effects may bring a scare,
Like **flushing, dyspnea, chest pressure**, rare.
Bradycardia, asystole for a beat or two—
It's short-lived, but still can spook you.

Nurses, prep and act with speed,
This drug works fast—**you must proceed**
With IV push in **1-2 seconds**, tight—
Follow with a flush, and hold on tight!
Place the patient on the **ECG**,
And watch that blip—it's supposed to be.
Continuous monitoring is a must,
And **crash cart ready**, just in trust.
Teach the patient what they'll feel—
A **brief pause**, then back to real.
It might feel like their heart gave out,
But reassure—no need to doubt.
No **black box warning**, but caution still:
In **asthma**, may cause **bronchospasm** ill.
Use lower dose if on **dipyridamole**,
And **theophylline** may block its role.
Interacts with caffeine and such,
So **methylxanthines** may weaken its touch.
Carbamazepine? Slows heart more—
So monitor close, that's what it's for.
Adenosine, so short, so bold,
A rapid push, and then behold.
Reset the heart, like flipping a switch—
But only if you **act fast and pitch.**

ALBUMIN
(ALBUMINAR, ALBUTEIN)
Plasma Volume Expander / Colloid

Albumin, drawn from human blood,
Restores the volume like a flood.
A **colloid**, not a crystallo-salt,
It **pulls fluid in**—a strong osmotic vault.
It **increases oncotic pressure** fast,
So fluid in tissues doesn't last.
It **shifts the fluid to intravascular space**,
Bringing back volume to stabilize pace.
Used for **hypovolemia** that's severe,
Shock, **burns**, and **liver failure** clear.
Hypoalbuminemia, third-spacing too—
It helps the **BP** climb back through.
But side effects can still arise:
Fever, rash, or **flushing thighs**,
Chills, tachycardia, or worse, **pulmonary edema**—
Watch their lungs and keep your schema.

Nursing considerations to heed:
Use a **vented IV set** for speed.
Give it **slow**, don't rush the stream,
And **warm the vial**—don't cause a scream.
Monitor for **vitals, lungs, and I&Os**,
Watch for **fluid overload** as it flows.
Hemoglobin and hematocrit may shift—
So track labs closely, that's your gift.

Teach patients what's being done—
It's **pooled from plasma**, not just one.
Check **religious beliefs** as well—
Some may **refuse blood products**, do tell.
Though **no black box warning** appears,
Still screen for **clots or allergy fears**.
And if they have **anemia** or **HF**,
Use caution—**don't overload** their shelf.
May **interact with ACE inhibitors**, slight—
Cause **hypotension**, if not done right.
So hold them briefly, just in case,
And check the patient's **hydration base**.
Albumin, rich and tightly bound,
Can turn things fast when low's been found.
A plasma hero, drawn with care—
Just monitor well and stay aware.

AMIODARONE (CORDARONE, PACERONE)

Antiarrhythmic - Class III Potassium Channel Blocker

When **heartbeats race** or skip their song,
Amiodarone comes strong and long.
It blocks those **potassium channels** tight,
To help the rhythm beat just right.
Used in **V-tach** and **V-fib** fast,
And **A-fib** when it's beating past.
It **slows conduction**, **lengthens repolarization**,
To calm the heart's wild excitation.

But nurses, hear this **urgent tale**—
Side effects may tip the scale:
Pulmonary fibrosis, **hepatotoxicity**,
And **thyroid shifts**—both high and low, you see.
Watch for **blue-gray skin**, a **visual haze**,
Corneal deposits may cloud their gaze.
Bradycardia, **hypotension**, too,
Especially when the IV's in view.

Monitor ECGs on repeat,
And **pulmonary scans** if lungs feel beat.
Check **liver labs**, and **thyroid tests**,
And **eye exams** to rule out stress.
Teach patients, "No **grapefruit juice**, please,"
It messes with metabolism ease.
And warn of **photosensitivity**—
The sun may cause skin injury.

Black Box Warnings are not few:
For **lungs, liver, thyroid**, it warns you true.
Long-term use? Proceed with care,
And always **document** what you prepare.
Interacts with **digoxin, warfarin**, too—
Both levels rise, so watch what you do.
Also **beta-blockers, CCBs**—
Can lower heart rate dangerously.

It's potent, complex, used with skill,
In codes or rhythms standing still.
But nurse, take caution every day
With **Amiodarone**, and guide the way.

ANGIOTENSIN II (GIAPREZA)

Vasopressor – Synthetic Angiotensin II

In **shock** where pressure's dropping low,
Giapreza helps that pressure grow.
A **vasopressor** strong and new,
It mimics what the body **can't quite do**.
It's **Angiotensin II**, you see—
A **RAAS hormone** synthetically.
It **tightens vessels**, boosts **MAP** fast,
When others fail, it holds you last.

Used in **septic** or **distributive shock**,
When **norepinephrine** fails to rock.
It gets infused through **central line**,
Titrated slow, then held in line.
Watch for **thromboembolic risk**,
DVTs can form and twist.
Also **headache, fever**, pain at site,
And **peripheral ischemia** just might bite.

Monitor **MAP**, and perfusion glow—
Are **kidneys working**, urine flow?
Check for **clots**, and **limb discoloration**,
It's not a med for hesitation.
No **Black Box Warning**, but beware—
Thrombosis risk is always there.
So **VTE prophylaxis** should align
Before you start that pressure climb.

Don't mix with **ACE inhibitors**,
Or **ARBs**—they're **receptor blockers**.
They counteract and block the way
That **Giapreza** must act today.
Tell the team to **watch the line**,
And assess **peripheral perfusion** time.
For patients deep in **hypotense**,
This drug may be the last defense.

It's not for every BP low—
But in a crash, it's good to know.
One final press to bring them through,
Angiotensin II, tried and true.

ASPIRIN (ASA)
Antiplatelet - NSAID - Salicylate

Aspirin's small but mighty still,
It **blocks COX enzymes**—that's the skill.
It stops **thromboxane**, clears the slate,
So **platelets** won't coagulate.
It's used to **thin the blood**, prevent **MI**, **stroke**, and **cardiac event**.
It's also used for **pain** and **fever**,
And **inflammation** in any lever.

Side effects? Don't turn your back—
GI bleeding, **tinnitus**, attack.
Reye's syndrome risk in kids is high,
So never give when flu is nigh.
Ulcers, **bruising**, **nausea**, too,
Hives, **asthma**, if allergic crew.
And watch the dose in renal strain—
It may increase the **kidney pain**.

Monitor for **bleeding signs**,
Black stools, or gums between the lines.
Check for **ringing in the ears**,
A classic sign when **toxicity nears**.
Teach them **take with food or milk**,
To keep the gut lining smooth as silk.
Hold before surgery, five to seven days,
To minimize blood loss in surgical phase.

There's a **Black Box Warning**, it's not mild—
GI risk and **bleeds** that can get wild.
And **NSAID combo** ups that game—
So be cautious if they're in the same.
It **interacts** with many meds:
Anticoagulants, **steroids**, **NSAIDs**.
It raises **bleed risk**, lowers platelets more,
So drug review is key before.

A classic med that still holds weight,
When given smart, it works real great.
So **Aspirin** earns respect each day,
Just keep the risks in firm display.

ATROPINE (ATROPEN)
Anticholinergic - Muscarinic Antagonist

Atropine blocks the **vagus nerve**,
So heartbeats rise and lungs can serve.
It **blocks acetylcholine** with might,
To stop **parasympathetic** fight.
It treats a heart that's beating slow—
Bradycardia, with a low flow.
Also used in **organophosphate tox**,
And **pupil dilation** in eye docs.

Watch for signs that quickly show:
Dry mouth, blurry vision, go slow.
Urine retention, hot, dry skin,
And **constipation** from within.
The classic signs? Easy to recite:
Can't pee, can't see, can't spit, can't... fight!
(Well, **poop**, but we keep it clean—
You get the gist of what we mean.)

Monitor **HR** and **ECG**,
It may make **tachycardia** be.
In high doses, CNS goes wild—
Confusion, restlessness, not mild.
Teach them it may cause **light sensitivity**,
So wear those shades with some humility.
Don't mix it with **antihistamines**,
Or **tricyclics**—those **dry effects** are mean.

No Black Box Warning, but still beware—
It's strong and fast, so nurses care.
Especially in the **elderly**,
Where **delirium** can quickly be.
Used in **codes** or for **eye exams**,
Or to treat **toxic nerve agent jams**.
When **cholinergic storm** is near,
Atropine is the med we cheer.

CLEVIDIPINE (CLEVIPREX)

Antihypertensive – Dihydropyridine Calcium Channel Blocker

Clevidipine, smooth and slick,
Drops BP down—and does it quick.
A **calcium channel blocker** class,
It works in **arteries**, not the gas.
It blocks **calcium influx** at the gate,
So **vasodilation** can regulate.
Used in **hypertensive crises** fast,
Especially when a **surgery's** cast.

It's **IV only, short half-life**,
Perfect for **tight BP** in strife.
Titrated drip, not pushed or slammed—
This one's **precise**, not one to jam.
Watch for **reflex tachycardia**,
And sometimes **nausea, fever aura**.
Hypotension, headache, dizzy cue,
Can come on fast—observe the crew.

Monitor the **BP closely**, friend,
Both **systolic** and **diastolic trend**.
Check **heart rate** too—can quickly climb,
As vessels dilate over time.
Contraindicated in **soy or egg** allergy,
Since it's in a **lipid emulsion**, see.
And don't mix in the same IV line
With other meds—keep flow just fine.

No Black Box Warning, but here's the tip:
Discard **after 12 hours** from the drip.

Strict aseptic technique's your guide—
To keep infection risk denied.
No **oral form**, and **not for chronic**,
This med's for **acute BP tectonic**.
It acts like **nicardipine**, but faster—
In pressure storms, it's the master.

Clevidipine—short, controlled, and neat,
Keeps crashing pressure on its feet.
Just keep your monitor and math on deck,
To steer this ship without a wreck.

DILTIAZEM (CARDIZEM)
Calcium Channel Blocker - Non-Dihydropyridine

Diltiazem slows the rhythm down,
For hearts that **race and pound around**.
A **calcium channel blocker** strong,
That keeps the **rate and rhythm** long.
It **blocks calcium** in the heart and vessels,
So **afterload** and **contractility** settle.
Used in **A-fib**, **SVT**, **hypertension**,
And **angina** with heart tension.
It's a **non-dihydropyridine**—
It calms the **rate** where **nodes convene**.
Negative inotrope, watch the squeeze,
Too much can **drop the heart with ease**.
Side effects you must catch:
Bradycardia, **hypotension** batch.
Dizziness, **flushing**, and **headache** rise,
And **edema** under the eyes.

Monitor **EKG** and **BP flow**,
Check for **heart blocks** that may show.
It may worsen **CHF**, be warned,
If **ejection fraction's** already scorned.
Hold the med if pulse is slow—
Below **60**, let the provider know.
Same for **BP** under **90 systolic**,
That drop can turn the shift symbolic.

It **interacts** with **beta-blockers**,
And **digoxin**—both **rhythm shockers**.
Watch **liver enzymes**, monitor labs,
And teach them to avoid **grapefruit scabs**.
No **Black Box Warning**, but it's a star
In managing hearts from near to far.
Still, use caution with **renal disease**,
And keep an eye on **CHF with ease**.
Teach them: rise **slowly** from the bed,
Dizzy spells may hit the head.
And don't stop **abruptly**, friend—
The rebound rate may ascend.
Diltiazem—for hearts that fly,
To bring that rhythm back to sky.
With careful checks and knowledge clear,
This med brings calm from rate to fear.

DIGOXIN (LANOXIN)
Cardiac Glycoside - Positive Inotrope, Negative Chronotrope

Digoxin helps the **heart beat strong**,
But too much can go very wrong.
It gives the **myocardium power**,
While making **heartbeats slow and lower**.
It's used in **heart failure, A-fib,** too—
To help the rhythm stay **steady and true**.
It boosts **contractility** so well,
And **slows conduction** through the **AV shell**.
But here's the catch: it's got a range—
Therapeutic but **tight and strange**.
0.5 to 2.0 is the goal,
Above that, it can take a toll.
Signs of **toxicity** are key—
Blurred vision, nausea, halos you see.
Bradycardia, dizzy, not quite right?
Check that level—day or night.
Watch **K+ levels** closely, friend—
Hypokalemia brings a dangerous end.
It makes the **myocardium twitch**,
And worsens **dig toxicity** quick.
Apical pulse—you must assess!
For **one full minute**, nonetheless.
Hold the dose if **pulse drops low**—
Below **60**, let the prescriber know.
It **interacts** with many meds—
Like **diuretics**, which mess with **electrolyte threads**.

Amiodarone, verapamil, too,
May raise **dig levels** out of the blue.
No **Black Box Warning**, but it's old school—
And needs a **nurse who knows the rule**.
Taught in **checklists**, tested lots—
Because **digoxin** can connect or clot.
Teach patients not to skip or stack,
And take it daily—**never backtrack**.
Watch for signs the dose is steep,
And always **store the med out of reach**.
Digoxin—slow and steady heart,
But know the signs before you start.
With labs and checks, you'll give it right,
And help their heart beat with more might.

DOBUTAMINE

Dobutamine gets the heart to rise,
With **stronger beats** but no surprise.
It's a **beta-1 selective friend**,
Used when **cardiac output** needs to mend.
It boosts **contractility**, not rate,
Though **tachycardia** can still create.
Used in **heart failure, cardiogenic shock**,
To get that **circulation out of lock**.

Given by **IV**, in drips it flows,
Titrated as the **monitor shows**.
Acts fast—but **short-lived**, too,
So watch the rhythm as you do.
Side effects you must prepare:
Increased heart rate, BP scare.
Can cause **angina, palpitations**,
And rare **arrhythmic fluctuations**.

Watch for signs the heart's too taxed,
Like **chest pain** or **oxygen relaxed**.
Monitor **EKG** and **output stats**,
And keep an eye for **PVC spats**.
It **interacts** with drugs like **MAOIs**,
Which may make pressure **quickly rise**.
Also use with care in **Afib cases**,
Since it may **increase conduction paces**.

No Black Box Warning, but handle tight—
Not for every failing fight.
Avoid in **hypovolemia's zone**,
Fill the tank before it's shown.

Teach: This drug's **short-term support**,
In ICU or **cardiac transport**.
It won't fix hearts that **need repair**,
But gives them time to breathe some air.

Dobutamine—with focused plan,
Supports the beat, as best it can.
With pumps and charts and eyes that scan,
The nurse ensures the heart can stand.

DOPAMINE (INTROPIN)
Inotrope & Vasopressor - Adrenergic Agonist

Dopamine—a dose-defined star,
Works **differently** depending how far.
It stimulates **dopamine, beta,** and **alpha,** too,
Each at its dose—so monitor through!
At **low dose** (1-5 mcg/kg/min),
It **boosts renal perfusion** from within.
It opens up the **kidneys' gate**,
To help with **urine output rate**.
At **moderate dose** (5-10 range),
It's **beta-1** that takes the stage.
Increased contractility and **heart's beat**,
Help **cardiac output** stay on its feet.
At **high dose** (10+ mcg/kg/min),
It turns **vasopressor** to win.
Alpha-1 kicks in, tightens the squeeze,
To raise **BP** and **vessel ease**.

Used for **shock, HF,** and **low perfusion**,
But must be used with close inclusion.
IV only, on a **pump it drips**,
And always through **central line tips**.
Side effects? Be on alert:
Tachycardia, palpitations that hurt.
Angina, necrosis, if IV leaks—
Extravasation is what no one seeks.
So monitor **site** and **flow real close**,
And keep **phentolamine** for the dose.

It's the **antidote** if tissues burn—
Injected fast, it helps them turn.
No Black Box Warning, but proceed with skill,
This drug is strong and **dose-level will**.
Correct hypovolemia first,
Or Dopamine's effect is cursed.
Teach the team: don't let it run
Without the checks—it's not for fun.
Vitals, **urine output**, and **EKG**,
All must be watched continuously.
Dopamine—complex, layered, wise,
But with good hands, it stabilizes.
In crash or code, it holds the line,
A lifeline drip, in rhythmic time.

EPHEDRINE
Adrenergic Agonist - Sympathomimetic

Ephedrine gives the system a jolt,
A **sympathomimetic** with lightning bolt.
It works on **alpha and beta alike**,
To boost the **BP**, **HR**, and strike.
It stimulates **norepinephrine** flow,
To raise **BP** when it drops too low.
Used in **anesthesia-induced hypotension**,
And sometimes **bronchospasm** prevention.

It's also used for **nasal congestion**,
Though now with limits due to tension.
(Over-the-counter? It's rarely found—
Thanks to rules that keep it bound.)
Side effects race with heart in tow:
Tachycardia, **palpitations** grow.
Anxiety, **tremor**, **urinary retention**,
And **hypertension** may get attention.

It's given **IV**, sometimes **IM**,
Monitor **BP**, keep **EKG** in trim.
Can cross the **BBB** just fine,
Causing **CNS effects** in line.
No Black Box Warning, but still proceed,
With caution for those with **heart disease**.
Avoid in **angina**, **arrhythmias**, too,
Or **hyperthyroidism**—it may overdo.

Watch for **urinary retention signs**,
Especially in men with **prostate lines**.
It can **interact** with **MAOIs**,
Causing pressure spikes to the skies.
Also avoid with **beta-blockers**,
They may reduce the pressor shockers.
And take care in **elderly** use,
As **CNS stimulation** might let loose.

Ephedrine—fast, short, and bold,
But nursing hands must take the hold.
A **rescue med**, not for long play,
Used with skill, it saves the day.

EPINEPHRINE (ADRENALIN)

Adrenergic Agonist - Alpha & Beta Agonist (Sympathomimetic)

Epinephrine, fierce and fast,
A **rescue med** that's built to last.
It hits **alpha**, **beta-1**, and **beta-2**,
For emergencies coming through.
Used for **anaphylaxis** first in line,
It opens airways **just in time**.
Also used in **asystole**,
Shock, asthma, and **bradycardic roles**, you see.
It **vasoconstricts** with **alpha might**,
To raise the **BP** back to right.
Then **beta-1** boosts **heart rate and squeeze**,
While **beta-2** brings **bronchodilation ease**.
Can be given **IM**, **IV**, or **ET tube**,
Or **subQ** depending on the move.
In **codes**, it's given **every 3–5 min**,
Until the heart comes back again.
Side effects? They come with speed:
Tachycardia, hypertension, sweat, tremble, need.
Restlessness, angina, palpitations,
Even **V-fib** in rare situations.
Monitor ECG, vitals tight,
And always prep for **cardiac fright**.
Can raise **glucose, lactic acid**, too,
So labs may change as rescue's due.
Teach for **EpiPen** with clear view:
Thigh injection, hold for **ten**, not two.
Always **call 911** post-shot,
One dose may not be all they've got.

Black Box Warning doesn't apply,
But still, it's strong—respect it high.
Avoid if **MAOIs** are near,
They **amplify effects**—a serious fear.
Beta-blockers may blunt the thrill,
Making **epi less effective still**.
And **inhaled anesthetics** may ignite
A **dysrhythmia**—not a light fright.
Epinephrine—a med that saves,
Through codes, **anaphylaxis waves**.
Fast and potent, small but grand,
In the right nurse's steady hand.

ESMOLOL (BREVIBLOC)
Beta Blocker - Beta-1 Selective (Cardioselective)

Esmolol—a heart's reset,
A **beta-1 blocker** fast and wet.
Used when rhythms **run too high**,
It helps the **tachycardia** die.
It slows the **SA and AV node**,
To bring the **rate** back down the road.
Used in **SVT**, and **A-fib** fast,
And **hypertensive crisis** that won't pass.

It's **IV only**, short half-life,
Ideal for **emergency cardiac strife**.
Titrated drip, **on a pump**, precise,
With **rapid onset**—cool as ice.
Side effects are mostly tame,
But nurses still must **watch the game**:
Bradycardia, hypotension,
Heart block, fatigue, and **cool skin tension.**

May also mask **hypoglycemia signs**,
So caution with **diabetic lines**.
It's cardioselective, but not 100%—
So **asthmatics** may still feel the event.
Monitor ECG, BP, and **rate**,
Especially if rhythms fluctuate.
Taper slow if ending the med—
Or **rebound tachy** may raise its head.

No Black Box Warning, but use wise,
In **CHF**, it may compromise.
Contraindicated in **heart block degree**,
Or if **sinus brady** comes to be.
Teach the team to check **apical pulse**,
Before each change or dosing impulse.
And **don't give with other AV-slowing drugs**,
Like **verapamil**—they may hug.

Esmolol—a beta breeze,
To bring the **racing heart some ease**.
Short-acting, strong, and sharply led,
In the right hands, it keeps hearts fed.

HYDRALAZINE (APRESOLINE)
Antihypertensive - Direct-Acting Vasodilator

Hydralazine, a pressure dropper,
Works on **arteries**, not the stopper.
It causes **vasodilation wide**,
So **afterload** takes quite a slide.
Used for **hypertension** hard to tame,
And **pre-eclampsia** stakes its claim.
Also for **heart failure** in select care,
When other meds can't quite get there.

It's **oral or IV**—short-acting thrill,
Great for a **rapid pressure spill**.
But monitor close with every dose,
Because **reflex tachycardia** can impose.
Side effects to watch and say:
Dizziness, **headache**, every day.
Flushing, **palpitations**, too,
And **edema** that may come through.

Long-term use may rarely bring,
A **lupus-like syndrome**—chronic sting.
Look for **joint pain**, **fever**, **fatigue**,
ANA test may show the league.
No Black Box Warning, but caution deep—
In **renal patients**, watch labs keep.
Avoid abrupt stops in the plan,
Or **BP spikes** may quickly span.

Teach: Rise **slowly**, don't rush to stand,
Or **orthostatic** drops may land.
Check **heart rate**, **BP** each day,
And log those numbers on the way.
It works well with **beta-blockers**, too,
To tame the **tachy** rushing through.
Also paired with **diuretics** fair,
To handle **fluid buildup** there.

Hydralazine—arterial grace,
Bringing **blood pressure** back to place.
With **monitoring**, **labs**, and nursing flair,
You'll guide each dose with expert care.

ISOPROTERENOL (ISUPREL)

Beta Adrenergic Agonist – Non-Selective (1 & 2)

Isoproterenol, beta boost,
A **non-selective** beta host.
It hits both **beta-1** and **beta-2**,
To get the heart and lungs **in view**.
Beta-1 kicks the **heart rate up**,
In **bradycardia** or when rhythms disrupt.
It increases **contractility**,
And **cardiac output** flows more free.

Beta-2 opens up the air,
So **bronchodilation** clears the air.
Used in **heart blocks, shock,** and **asthma past**,
Though newer meds have outpaced fast.
IV or IM, sometimes **subQ**,
This med works fast and pulls them through.
It's short in half-life—**minutes few**,
So continuous drips are common too.

Side effects? They're often bold:
Tachycardia, palpitations take hold.
Angina, tremors, nervous feel,
And **hypotension** may sneak in the deal.
Monitor **HR, BP,** and **EKG**,
This med can cause **dysrhythmia spree**.
Caution in **CAD, angina pain**,
Too much push can **strain the brain**.

No Black Box Warning, but know this truth—
It's rarely used in modern youth.
Reserved for cases **drug-resistant**,
Or when other **inotropes** are distant.
Watch for **hypokalemia**, too,
From **shifting K+** the beta way through.
And monitor **glucose**, it may rise,
So diabetics need nursing eyes.

Isoproterenol—a rare, strong spark,
For rhythms lost or lungs too dark.
With pumps, monitors, and steady hand,
You'll guide its use just as planned.

ISOSORBIDE DINITRATE
Nitrate - Antianginal Vasodilator

Isosorbide dinitrate, a nitrate class name, Relaxes smooth vessels to help chest pain. By reducing preload and afterload strain, It eases the heart's work and vascular pain.

It **dilates the veins** and **coronary flow**, So **angina pain** has no room left to grow. It's used for **chronic stable angina** relief, And **heart failure** patients may also find peace.

Take it **sublingual**, oral, or patch— The **onset is slower** than nitro's quick catch. It's **longer-acting**, so don't be confused— For **prevention**, not rescue, this one is used.

A **major risk** is **orthostatic low BP**, So rise up **slowly** and move carefully. A **nitrate headache** may come on strong, But it's common— and won't last long.

Watch for **flushing**, **dizziness**, or **blurred sight**, And report **fainting** or palpitations at night. **Avoid alcohol**—it worsens the dip, And always sit down if you feel yourself slip.

Sildenafil and nitrates should never combine— The **BP will crash** and you'll flatline in time. Ask men discreetly 'bout **ED pills** they take, It could save their life for their nitrate's sake.

Nitrate tolerance can happen too— So your dosing schedule should split the view. Allow **nitrate-free hours** each day or night, To keep the med working just right.

Monitor BP before each dose, Hold if **hypotension** is too close. Check **HR and chest pain pattern** as well— Is it **improving**, or hard to quell?

If using patches, **rotate the site**, And **remove before bed**, unless told it's right. Teach them the difference between **rescue and daily**, And carry nitro for chest pain that flares up acutely.

Contraindicated in recent MI, If **severe anemia** or shock is nearby. It's also not safe with **glaucoma** flare— Too much pressure is a risk in there.

With heart meds, teach them the plan: What to **expect**, and how to **scan** For signs of **hypotension**, or worse distress— And to call for help when symptoms progress.

So teach with care and check those signs, Track the **angina**, and set clear lines. For long-term pain, this med's your mate— It's **Isosorbide Dinitrate**.

LEVOSIMENDAN
Inotropic Agent (Calcium Sensitizer & Potassium Channel Opener)

When the **heart can't pump**, and **failure is near**,
Levosimendan may bring back some cheer.
It **boosts contraction**—a cardiac lift,
But does it gently, like a gifted shift.
It **sensitizes troponin** to **calcium's touch**,
So the **heart beats stronger**, but not too much.
It opens **potassium channels** to **dilate**,
Reducing the strain on the vascular gate.

Given **IV in hospitals**, often in shock,
For **acute heart failure**—a ticking clock.
It helps the **left ventricle** pump with might,
While lowering **afterload**, keeping things light.
No **beta-blockade**, no increase in O₂ need,
It helps the heart pump without making it speed.
But watch for **hypotension**, or **headache**, or more,
And **arrhythmias** knocking at the ICU door.

It's not for the **long term**, or outpatient care,
Just for **crisis support** when the heart's in despair.

No U.S. approval (as of now, still debated),
But in Europe and others, it's often slated.
Check **electrolytes**, especially **potassium low**,
Watch for **QT prolongation**—a dangerous show.
Renal function needs watching, too,
And **liver metabolism** plays a role in what it'll do.

So **Levosimendan**, not yet widespread,
But in failing hearts, it may tread.
A helper in crisis, with power and grace,
Strengthening the beat while easing the race.

METOPROLOL (LOPRESSOR)
Beta Blocker - Beta-1 Selective (Cardioselective)

Metoprolol, calm and slow,
A **beta-1 blocker** in the flow.
It **slows the heart**, reduces strain,
Brings down **BP** and **chest pain**.
Used in **hypertension, MI,
Heart failure**, and **HRs too high**.
Also treats **angina** flare,
And **migraine prevention** here and there.
It blocks the **beta-1 receptor line**,
To drop the **rate** and **contractile spine**.
That means **less oxygen demand**,
A gift to hearts that can't withstand.
Side effects? There are a few:
Bradycardia, fatigue in view.
Hypotension, dizziness, cold hands,
And sometimes **heart block** where it stands.

Black Box Warning must be said:
Taper slowly—or risk the dread
Of **angina worsening** or **MI**,
If stopped abruptly, patients could die.
Watch for **blood sugar masking signs**,
In **diabetics**, it blurs the lines.
It hides the **tachy** that says "I'm low,"
So teach them other signs to know.
Check **apical pulse** before each dose,
If it's **under 60**, hold it close.

Same goes if **BP's too low**,
And notify the doc, you know.
Can be **IV push** in acute MI,
But mostly **oral** as days go by.
May be extended-release (Toprol XL),
So don't **crush or chew**—it won't go well.
Teach: Take it at the **same time each day**,
And rise up slow so you don't sway.
Avoid **alcohol** and **hot showers**, too—
They drop your pressure out of the blue.
Metoprolol—a cardio chill,
But takes a nurse with focused will.
With checks, teaching, and steady pace,
You'll guide this med with heart and grace.

MILRINONE (PRIMACOR)
Inotrope – Phosphodiesterase-3 Inhibitor

Milrinone, a cardiac lift,
Gives the **failing heart** a gift.
It's a **PDE-3 inhibitor** rare,
That boosts the **pump** and **vascular repair**.
Used in **heart failure**—acute and tight,
When the heart can't squeeze with might.
Increases **contractility** and **relaxation**,
While causing **vasodilation**.
It's given **IV**, slow and clear,
Often in ICU, with nurses near.
Short term use—**bridge to transplant**,
Or when other meds just can't.
Side effects to watch with speed:
Ventricular arrhythmias may take the lead.
Also **hypotension**, **headache**, signs
That **electrolytes** are crossing lines.
Check **potassium**, **platelets**, too,
And **renal function** must be in view.
Since it's cleared through **kidneys fast**,
Adjust the dose when GFR won't last.
No Black Box Warning, but don't relax—
It can still cause **sudden cardiac cracks**.
So **monitor ECG**, **vitals** on screen,
And have **rescue meds** on the scene.

It **increases CO**, drops **afterload**,
But may speed the heart down risky road.
So in **atrial fib**, watch it tight,
It might flip rhythms overnight.
Not for **chronic use** on home ground—
Too many risks the studies found.
But in the **hospital**, it earns its stay,
To keep the heart from slipping away.

Milrinone—a final spark,
For failing hearts lost in the dark.
With nurse-led care and constant check,
It gives the beat one last good trek.

NICARDIPINE (CARDENE)

Antihypertensive - Calcium Channel Blocker (Dihydropyridine)

Nicardipine, smooth and sleek,
A **calcium blocker** for pressure peaks.
It **relaxes arteries**, drops the load,
So **BP falls** on a smoother road.
Used for **hypertensive crisis** scenes,
Or **stroke care** when pressure leans.
Also helps with **angina** pain,
By letting oxygen freely reign.
It blocks the **L-type calcium gate**,
So **vascular smooth muscles** dilate.
But it doesn't hit the **heart too hard**,
Just vessels—so it's the BP guard.
IV drip is the common route,
In **ICU** or when things are acute.
Titrate slowly, watch the tone,
And **never give by IM** zone.
Side effects to watch with care:
Hypotension, headache, flushing flare.
Tachycardia may come in fast,
As **reflex beats** try to hold it last.
Check for **edema**, especially legs,
And **dizziness** if pressure begs.
Also **nausea, palpitations**, slight,
So stay alert throughout the night.
No Black Box Warning, but be wise—
Monitor BP and watch the size
Of **IV site** for any pain,
As **infiltration** brings tissue strain.
Caution in patients with **CHF**,
As fluid buildup may take a breath.
And avoid **grapefruit juice** in play—
It can mess how enzymes clear the way.
Teach: This med may cause a flush,
But it's not a reason for patient rush.
Rise up slow, and change positions light,
To avoid a **hypotensive fright**.

Nicardipine—a pressure guide,
That helps the vessels open wide.
With nursing care and drip control,
You'll guide this med to meet its goal

45

NIMODIPINE
Calcium Channel Blocker - Dihydropyridine (Cerebral Vasodilator)

Nimodipine, a niche delight,
Cerebral vessels—that's its fight.
A **calcium blocker**, smooth and clean,
It's used for **subarachnoid bleed** on scene.
Not for **BP** in the common way,
But to keep **vasospasms** far at bay.
It **dilates brain arteries**, nice and slow,
So oxygen-rich blood can freely flow.

Used in **aneurysmal hemorrhage**, post-rupture days,
To help prevent **ischemic phase**.
Given **oral**, or **NG/OG tube** with care,
But **never IV—severe risk** is there.
Side effects can still appear:
Hypotension, **bradycardia** near.
Also **flushing**, **nausea**, **dizzy head**,
So keep the patient safely in bed.

Black Box Warning shouts aloud:
Do NOT give IV—it's not allowed!
Cardiovascular collapse is the fear,
So double-check the route is clear.
Monitor **BP**, **HR**, and **neuro signs**,
As brain perfusion walks fine lines.
And if they're on for **21 days**,
Document those neuro-focused plays.

No grapefruit juice, that's a must—
It **raises levels**, breaks your trust.
And always check for **swallowing trouble**,
Crush it only if guidelines double.
Teach: This med's for **brain not chest**,
It helps the **vessels rest and rest**.
And though the BP may go low,
It's the **brain protection** that we show.

Nimodipine—a narrow scope,
But gives the brain a fighting hope.
With **timing**, **route**, and nurse command,
You'll help this med do what it's planned.

NITROGLYCERIN (NITROSTAT, TRIDIL)

Antianginal - Nitrate Vasodilator

Nitroglycerin, fast and slick,
Relieves **chest pain** mighty quick.
A **nitrate** that helps the vessels chill,
So **oxygen demand** goes downhill.
Used for **angina, MI**, and more,
Heart failure when the lungs feel sore.
It **dilates veins** to ease preload strain,
And opens arteries to soothe the pain.
Forms include **sublingual, IV, patch,**
Spray, ointment—there's quite a batch.
Sublingual tab is first to reach,
Place under tongue, let it breach.
Onset fast, like 1-3 mins,
But **IV drip** is used when the crisis begins.
Patch or ointment? Use with grace—
Rotate the **sites**, give **nitrate-free space**.
Side effects are often loud:
Headache, flushing, pressure downed.
Orthostatic hypotension rise,
So teach to stand up slow and wise.
Reflex tachycardia may appear,
As the body fights to persevere.
And **dizziness, syncope** might ensue—
So fall precautions? Yes, that too.
Black Box Warning? Not on file,
But still, this med needs careful style.
Never use with **PDE-5** meds—
Like **Viagra**, or you'll risk the beds.
Profound hypotension is the fear,
So always screen before you steer.
Teach: 1 tab under tongue, then wait,
If pain persists—**call 9-1-1** straight.
May repeat every 5, up to three,
But **don't drive yourself**—let help be free.
Check **BP** before each dose,
If it's too low, the drip may close.
Wear **gloves for paste**—don't absorb,
This potent med can **numb the absorb**.
Nitroglycerin—chest pain's foe,
But only safe when nurses know.
With **timing, teaching**, and careful checks,
You'll guide the dose and guard the next.

NITROPRUSSIDE (NIPRIDE)

Antihypertensive - Direct Vasodilator

Nitroprusside, fast and clean,
Drops the pressure **in between**.
A **direct vasodilator** true,
That opens **arteries and veins** for you.
Used in **hypertensive crises** bold,
Or **acute heart failure** when BP's cold.
IV infusion is the only way,
It works **within seconds**, not delay.
It decreases **preload** and **afterload** tight,
So the heart can **pump with less fight**.
But with great power comes the test—
It needs **close monitoring**, nothing less.
Side effects you must expect:
Severe hypotension can come direct.
Also **flushing, dizziness, tachy** quick,
And **nausea** may join the trick.
The big one, though, is **cyanide tox**,
When the med breaks down outside the box.
It releases **cyanide ions** in the blood—
So dosing too long can cause a flood.
Black Box Warning is a must:
Cyanide poisoning if used in trust
Too long, too fast, without great care—
It's deadly if you're unaware.
Protect from **light**—it breaks down quick,
Use **foil wrap** or **darkened stick**.
And discard the **blue or brown**—
That color means it's breaking down.
Monitor **thiocyanate levels** long,
Especially in **renal impaired**—things go wrong.
Check **lactic acid, mental state**,
For signs of toxicity that can't wait.
Titrate slow, and **BP track**,
With **arterial line** or pressure pack.
Keep **telemetry** on their chest,
And **ICU-level care** for best.

Nitroprusside—a pressure dive,
But needs full skill to keep alive.
With light, labs, and nurse precision,
You'll lead this drip with wise decision.

NOREPINEPHRINE (LEVOPHED)

Vasopressor - Alpha & Beta-1 Adrenergic Agonist

Norepinephrine, strong and fast,
A **vasopressor** built to last.
Known as **Levophed** on the floor,
It **raises BP** when shock hits the core.
It hits **alpha-1** with vasoconstrict,
To make those **vessels squeeze real quick**.
Also stims the **beta-1 heart**,
To pump with strength and do its part.

Used in **septic shock**, and **low BP**,
To keep up **perfusion** and **MAP** you see.
It's **IV only**, **titrated slow**,
With **central line**—that's the go.
Side effects? There's quite a list:
Hypertension, tachycardia exist.
Also **arrhythmias, limb ischemia** dark,
If **extravasation** leaves its mark.

Black Box Warning—this one is real:
Tissue necrosis is the deal.
If it leaks into the skin,
It can **damage tissues deep within**.
Keep **phentolamine** close at hand,
To block the **alpha** if things go unplanned.
Infiltrate? Inject around the site—
Save the tissue, make it right.

Monitor **BP** every beat,
Titrate per protocol, don't skip a seat.
Watch **urine output, peripheral perfusion**,
And signs of **organ confusion**.
Don't give with **alkaline meds**,
They break it down and dull its threads.
And teach your team: it's not for mild—
This drug's for when the vitals go wild.

Norepinephrine—power in vein,
For when the body's circling the drain.
With **nurse precision, eyes alert**,
You'll guide this drip and guard from hurt.

PHENYLEPHRINE (NEO-SYNEPHRINE)
Vasopressor - Alpha-1 Adrenergic Agonist

Phenylephrine, alpha king,
Vasoconstriction is its thing.
It hits **alpha-1** with power and pride,
To make those **vessels clamp and guide**.
Used in **shock** when **BP's low**,
But **heart rate's fine**—that's good to know.
Also used in **nasal spray**,
To clear congestion right away.

In **ICU**, it's **IV drip**,
To keep **MAP** above the slipping tip.
In **anesthesia**, it may show,
To raise the **pressure** when it's low.
Side effects can come on quick:
Hypertension, **reflex bradycardia** kick.
Too much squeeze? You may see signs
Of **ischemia** in toes and lines.

No **beta action**, so the heart
Stays untouched in its rate chart.
Great for **tachy-shocky** scenes,
Where **norepi** would be too mean.
No Black Box Warning, but stay smart—
This drug still strains the **vessel heart**.
Watch for **headache, anxiety, pain**,
And IV site for **tissue strain**.

Watch for **extravasation risk**,
Though not as high as others brisk.
Still—**phentolamine** should be nearby,
If infiltration does apply.
In **nasal sprays**, teach with care:
Rebound congestion if over there.
Use for **3 days max**, no more,
Or stuffy nose will hit the floor.

Phenylephrine—a squeeze that saves,
In **shock, anesthesia**, nasal caves.
With nursing checks and steady hand,
You'll help this pressor safely stand.

PHENTOLAMINE

Alpha-Adrenergic Antagonist - Antihypertensive / Infiltration Antidote

Phentolamine, reversal champ,
Treats when **vessels** go into cramp.
An **alpha-blocker**, smooth and wide,
It lets the blood flow open wide.
Used for **vasopressor extravasation**,
To save the skin from **necrotic devastation**.
Also used for **pheochromocytoma**,
To block the surge of **catecholoma**.
It **blocks alpha-1 receptors** fast,
So **vasoconstriction** doesn't last.
Drops **BP** in hypertensive tide,
From tumors or **clonidine withdrawal** side.
Given IV or **infiltrated near**,
Where **vasopressors** cause the fear.
Like **norepinephrine**, when it leaks,
This drug prevents **black skin peaks**.
Side effects? There are a few:
Tachycardia, **hypotension** in view.
Dizziness, flushing, nasal stuff,
And **GI upset** if taken tough.
No Black Box Warning, but handle wise,
Because sudden drops may **compromise**.
So monitor **BP, pulse**, and **pain**,
Especially when **IV sites strain**.
When used for **infiltration woes**,
Inject around where the necrosis grows.
5–10 mg diluted slow,
Into **ischemic skin** to help blood flow.

It may also help in rare events,
Like **cocaine-induced hypertension tents**.
But most of all, it's known to be
Tissue's guard from vasopressor spree.
Teach the team: it works **on site**,
And doesn't need to circulate right.
Just **draw it up** and act with speed,
When **Levophed leaks**, this is what you need.
Phentolamine—a vessel save,
For **pressors** that try to misbehave.
With nursing care and sharp injection,
You'll guard the skin from bad direction.

PROCAINAMIDE (PRONESTYL)

Antiarrhythmic – Class Ia Sodium Channel Blocker

Procainamide, rhythm's friend,
Helps the heart **arrhythmias end**.
A **Class Ia** drug on the chart,
It **slows conduction** through the heart.
Blocks the **sodium channels** wide,
To **lengthen action potential's ride**.
Used for **SVT**, **VT**, and more,
Even for **atrial fib** restore.

Given **IV**, and sometimes **oral**,
But in emergencies, it's most floral.
It's second-line for **stable VT**,
When **amiodarone** isn't the key.
Side effects? There's quite a few:
Hypotension, **bradycardia**, too.
Can cause **QT prolongation**,
Leading to **torsades**—a bad situation.

May also bring **lupus-like signs**,
With **joint pain**, **fever**, crossing lines.
So check for **ANA** and watch for aches,
Butterfly rash or facial flakes.
Black Box Warning is clear and firm:
For **blood dyscrasias** that may squirm.
Can lead to **agranulocytosis**,
So check **CBCs** with cautious doses.

Also risk of **proarrhythmia** climb—
So monitor **ECG** all the time.
And if the **QRS widens too**,
The dose may be too much for you.
Check for **liver** and **renal function**,
It clears slow with organ malfunction.
And teach patients: rise up slow,
Orthostatic drops may show.

Procainamide—a rhythm tune,
But not a med to give too soon.
With **labs**, **telemetry**, and heart-smart care,
You'll help the beat stay strong and fair.

PROPRANOLOL (INDERAL)

Beta Blocker – Nonselective (Beta-1 & Beta-2 Antagonist)

Propranolol, a blocker wide,
Hits **beta-1** and **beta-2** with pride.
It slows the **heart** and calms the race,
Drops **BP** and keeps a steady pace.
Used for **hypertension**, **angina** strain,
Arrhythmias, and **migraine** pain.
Also helps with **anxiety's grip**,
And **essential tremor** in its trip.
Sometimes used post-**MI** event,
To reduce death with its intent.
And treats **thyroid storm** with grace—
It slows the heart in that fast-paced chase.
But since it's **nonselective**, hear this clear:
It blocks **lungs**, too—so **asthma**? Fear.
Bronchospasm risk is high,
So **COPD** folks may not qualify.

Side effects you need to chart:
Bradycardia, **fatigue**, and heavy heart.
Also **hypotension**, **dizzy spell**,
And sometimes **depression** may dwell.
Masks hypoglycemia signs—
No **tachy**, just fatigue lines.
So **diabetics** must take care,
To watch for lows that won't declare.
No Black Box Warning for this one,
But **sudden stop** should not be done.
May cause **angina** or **MI return**,
So **taper slowly**—that's your concern.
Check **apical pulse** before each dose,
If **under 60**, hold it close.
Same for **BP** that drops too far,
Let the doc know where things are.
Teach: Take it **same time every day**,
Don't skip or double—don't delay.
Avoid **alcohol**, rise up slow,
And keep **log of vitals** as they go.
Propranolol—a calm, slow tide,
That keeps the heart from going wide.
With **nurse-led care** and patient trust,
You'll dose this med the way you must.

RANOLAZINE (RANEXA)

Antianginal Agent - Late Sodium Channel Inhibitor

When classic nitrates just don't suffice, Ranolazine steps in to stabilize twice. It's an **antianginal**, not a vasodilator, Working in cells as a **late sodium blocker**.
It **reduces calcium** inside heart muscle walls, Helping it relax when the tension calls. This improves perfusion, lowers O_2 need, Without changing **HR or BP speed**.
It's used in **chronic angina control**, Especially when **beta-blockers** don't fill the role. Taken **orally**, usually **BID**, Extended-release to keep symptoms at bay.
Common side effects aren't extreme, But **dizziness, nausea**, or **constipation** may be seen. Some patients report a bit of **QT prolongation**, So be cautious in those with cardiac complication.
Baseline EKGs are a must to begin, And check again if symptoms spin. **Monitor QT**—especially if they start to faint, Or complain of feeling like they're going to faint.
It's **not for acute** chest pain relief, So don't reach for it when symptoms are brief. It's a **maintenance med**, so stay on track, Don't double doses if you're off your back.
Avoid in patients with **liver disease**, Or **renal impairment** if severe, please. It's metabolized by **CYP3A4**, So beware of meds that increase it more.
Antifungals, macrolides, and **HIV meds**, Could make levels soar above safe threads. So always scan the patient's list, Before this drug joins the mix.
Tell them to report **palpitations** or light head, Or if their chest pain worsens instead. Don't crush or chew this **extended pill**, Swallow it whole—it's built for the chill.
Watch when combining with **digoxin** or **statins**, Levels can climb and lead to problems happenin'. So adjust those doses if used as a pair— And warn them of **muscle pain** or **air hunger** flare.
It's not as well known, but **quite effective**, For **stable angina** that's grown reflective. If nitrates or blockers just won't do, Ranolazine could carry them through.
So teach with care, monitor wise, And flag that **QT** before it can rise. Not for a crisis, but for daily peace— Ranolazine brings angina relief.

VASOPRESSIN (PITRESSIN)

Antidiuretic Hormone (ADH Analog) - Vasopressor / Hormone Replacement

Vasopressin, steady and tight,
Brings the **blood pressure** back to height.
A **synthetic ADH** in play,
It tells the **kidneys**: "Don't pee away."
Used in **shock** that's **vasodilated**,
Like **septic** or **distributive** states debated.
Also used in **cardiac arrest**,
With **epinephrine**, it works best.
Treats **diabetes insipidus**, too,
When **ADH is missing** in the brew.
It tells the body, "Hold that water,"
So output stops like it ought to.
IV, **IM**, or **subQ** routes go,
In ICU, it's a **drip** that's slow.
With **continuous BP monitor**,
To avoid too much vascular conquer.
Side effects you need to know:
Hypertension, **bradycardia** show.
Water intoxication is a real fear—
Causes **hyponatremia** to appear.
Also watch for **angina**, **gut cramps**, tight,
And **skin necrosis** if dosed just right.
So check **IV site**, guard the vein,
Extravasation causes pain.
No Black Box Warning, but here's the thing:
This med can **raise BP like a spring**.
So in patients with **coronary risk**,
Go slow, go steady—never brisk.
Monitor **I&Os**, **sodium** labs,
Urine specific gravity grabs.
In **DI**, you want the pee to slow,
In **shock**, you want the BP to grow.
Teach your team: it's not for light,
This med demands a **monitor night**.
Cardiac, renal, and brain in mind,
As **perfusion pressure** gets refined.
Vasopressin—a pressor true,
But only safe when watched by you.
With **drips**, **labs**, and bedside smarts,
You'll guide this med with nursing hearts.

VERAPAMIL (CALAN, ISOPTIN)

Calcium Channel Blocker - Class IV
Antiarrhythmic / Antihypertensive

Verapamil, smooth and slow,
Blocks **calcium channels** to help blood flow.
A **Class IV antiarrhythmic** role,
It brings the **heart rate** under control.
Used for **hypertension** high,
Angina, a-fib, when rhythms fly.
Also treats **SVT** with might,
To slow the **AV node** and set things right.

Given **oral** or as **IV**,
But **IV form** needs nurse to see.
Monitor BP and **heart rate** close—
It might bring both down too low a dose.
Side effects? They may appear:
Bradycardia, and **hypotension** clear.
Constipation is also common,
Especially when doses keep bombin'.

No Black Box Warning, but here's the thing:
With **beta blockers**, don't let it swing.
Together they **slow conduction** deep,
And may cause **heart block** or a **brady creep**.
Use caution in **heart failure** state,
It may reduce that ejection rate.
Also watch **liver**—it clears the med,
So dose adjustments may be ahead.

Avoid **grapefruit juice** in meals,
It **inhibits enzymes**, messes deals.
And rise up slow—**orthostatic signs**
Can catch the unaware at times.
Teach to report **swelling, dizzy feel**,
And if their **heartbeat slows or reels**.
Take **with food** to guard the gut,
And don't stop suddenly—never abrupt.

Verapamil—a steady tide,
To help the heart and vessels glide.
With **rhythm checks** and nursing grace,
You'll keep this med in the safest place.

Part III
Thrombolytics, Anticoagulants & Reversal Agents

ALTEPLASE (ACTIVASE)
Thrombolytic - Tissue Plasminogen Activator (tPA)

Alteplase works to **break a clot**,
In strokes or MIs, it's used a lot.
It mimics **tPA**, our body's way
To **dissolve fibrin**—clears the way.
It turns on **plasmin**, which breaks down
The **fibrin mesh** that clots have found.
So blood can flow back through the vein,
And lessen tissue death and pain.

Used in **MI**, **stroke**, and **PE**,
But timing's key—**ASAP**.
Ischemic stroke? You've got three hours
To give the dose and save brain power.
Watch for **bleeding**, big and small—
Intracranial is worst of all.
Bruising, low BP, nausea, too,
May show that bleeding's breaking through.

Check recent **surgery**, wounds, or falls—
It's **contraindicated** in those calls.
Avoid **needle sticks** and things invasive,
Because this drug is **hemostasis-erasing**.
Monitor **INR** and **aPTT**,
And **hemoglobin** carefully.
Look for signs of **neuro change**,
A sudden shift can be quite strange.

Teach the team: **One IV line**,
Keep it clean and mark the time.
Vital signs must be **close and tight**,
For **bleeding risks** throughout the night.
Black Box Warning? There is none,
But don't relax—this drug can stun.
Drug interactions? Think with care—
Anticoagulants? Double beware.

This med's a **last chance** kind of dance,
To give a patient one more chance.
Handle gently, act with speed—
Alteplase meets urgent need.

ANDEXANET ALFA
Antidote - Factor Xa Inhibitor Reversal Agent

When bleeding won't stop and the pressure climbs, And the culprit is **rivaroxaban** or **apixaban**'s lines, Andexanet Alfa comes to the fight— A **Factor Xa antidote**, fast and right.

It works by **binding the Xa inhibitors** tight, Neutralizing their clot-busting might. A **recombinant decoy**—cleverly made, It mops up the meds so clotting's replayed. Use it in **life-threatening bleeds**, Like **GI hemorrhage** or urgent needs. It's given **IV**, with a **bolus then drip**, In trauma, stroke, or surgical slip.

Before you begin, check **coag labs** first, And monitor closely for **clotting reversed**. Watch for **DVT, PE**, or MI signs— Because clotting can surge as med declines.

This drug's **not for routine nosebleeds**, please— It's saved for **major bleeds** and crises. Use with caution and consult fast— This med is **costly**, and its effects don't last. Don't mix with **heparin**—it might **bind instead**, Neutralizing both and messing with the thread. And be cautious if **thrombosis history** is real— This reversal can **trigger a clotting ordeal**.

No food or pills interact directly, But warn them: side effects may come unexpectedly. **Flushing, nausea**, or **pneumonia signs**, And sometimes **UTIs** cross the lines.

Rebound anticoagulation may appear, So a new plan must be crystal clear. Restart anticoagulants when it's safe, Once the bleeding has left no trace. Document **reason**, **dose**, and **timing well**, Because in lawsuits, this med tends to dwell. And advise your patient why it's rare— Not a go-to for daily scare.

So when Factor Xa goes too far, And blood won't clot near vein or scar, Andexanet steps in—quick and clean— To halt the flood and intervene.

ARGATROBAN
Anticoagulant - Direct Thrombin Inhibitor

When **heparin** harms instead of heals, And **HIT** becomes a real ordeal, Argatroban enters with a brand-new plan— A **direct thrombin blocker**, no heparin in hand.

It **inhibits factor IIa** directly at site, Preventing clots from gaining their might. Used in **heparin-induced thrombocytopenia**, To stop the spread of thrombin-related anemia.

Also used in **PCI** when HIT is a risk, This med keeps platelets from joining the mix. It's **given IV**, with a **weight-based start**, And titrated slowly—it's not for the heart.

There's **no reversal**, so check it right— Monitor **aPTT** to prevent a fright. Keep levels **1.5 to 3 times the norm**, And adjust the drip if trends transform.

Bleeding is the primary threat, From gums to urine, or black-tarry sweat. So check for bruising, flank pain, or red streak, And hold the dose if the patient grows weak.

Unlike heparin, no antidote lies, So **monitor trends** and act if they rise. No need to monitor **platelets for HIT**, Because this drug is used **because** of it.

If the liver is weak, the dose may stay— **Argatroban's cleared the hepatic way**. No renal dosing is needed here, But in liver disease, go slow and steer.

Avoid combining with **antiplatelet crew**, Like clopidogrel or ASA too. The **bleed risk spikes** when both unite, So weigh your options—bleed or fight?

No food interactions you need to dread, But always check what's being fed. Avoid IM shots or risky pokes, And always use soft brushes, no jokes.

Warn them: **black stools, bloody noses, pink pee**— Are all red flags for an urgent plea. And in post-op patients or trauma cases, Bleeding could show in hidden spaces.

So when **HIT** has halted the heparin train, And clots are forming deep in the vein, Argatroban's your IV friend— Until the patient is safe again.

BIVALIRUDIN
Anticoagulant - Direct Thrombin Inhibitor

When clots are looming and time runs thin, You might reach for **Bivalirudin**. A **direct thrombin blocker**, like Argatroban's kin, Used in **PCI** to stop clots within.
It binds to **thrombin** and blocks its spark, Halting fibrin before it leaves a mark. No antithrombin needed—it works alone, A clean, **reversible**, **IV-only** zone.
Used when **heparin's not safe to use**, Like **HIT** or PCI where risk accrues. Especially helpful when **heparin failed**, Or bleeding risks have wildly scaled.
Start it **in the cath lab**, right on time, To prevent **stent thrombosis** down the line. No mixing errors, no platelets touched— It acts with purpose, not too much.
aPTT is the lab you'll trend, Though it's short-acting and may not extend. When drip stops flowing, it fades out fast, In **less than an hour**, its work has passed.
Cleared by the **kidneys**, so go slow with care If **renal function** is impaired there. Dose may be lowered or paused a beat, To avoid a bleed where vessels meet.
Bleeding is still your number-one fear— Gums, urine, stool—or a sudden smear. Hold pressure longer at IV sites, And avoid sharp tools or razors at night.
No **reversal agent** has been approved, But with short half-life, it's quickly removed. Just pause the drip if signs arise, And check labs closely before surprise.
It won't cause HIT—it's **HIT-safe gold**, But bleeding rules still must be told. Avoid combining with other thinners, Unless cardiology clears the winners.
Teach signs of **bleeding, bruising**, or pain, Especially post-PCI when pressure may strain. And no IM injections should ever be done— Use soft toothbrushes until bleeding risk is none.
So when thrombin is high and platelets align, But **heparin or warfarin** aren't the right line, **Bivalirudin** holds the clotting back— A clean, fast stop on the thrombin track.

CLOPIDOGREL (PLAVIX)
Antiplatelet – ADP Receptor Inhibitor

Clopidogrel, a platelet foe,
Helps keep **clots** from stealing the show.
It blocks **ADP receptor's seat**,
So platelets **can't aggregate or meet**.
Used for **MI**, **stroke**, and **stent protection**,
It **prevents thrombosis**, not infection.
Also used in **PAD**,
To keep those vessels flowing free.
Side effects you need to know:
Bleeding risk is first to show.
Bruising, epistaxis, GI pain,
And **rash** or **diarrhea** may remain.
Rare but real is **TTP**,
A **medical emergency** you must see:
Thrombocytopenia, anemia, clots—
Watch **neuro status**, urine spots.

No **antidote**—so act with speed
If **bleeding signs** or labs mislead.
Check **H&H, platelet counts**,
And **stool for blood** in small amounts.
Teach patients: **Don't stop on your own**,
Unless the prescriber makes it known.
Take it **daily, same time**—stick tight,
And **report any bleeding** out of sight.
Don't pair it up with **NSAID friends**,
Or **anticoagulants**—that risk extends.
Watch **omeprazole**, it may block
The liver enzyme **CYP2C19's clock**.
There **is a Black Box Warning** clear:
Some **can't metabolize** it well, we fear.
They're **"poor metabolizers"** with low effect—
So test if outcomes seem incorrect.
Used with **aspirin**, side by side,
For **dual antiplatelet** power ride.
It helps keep vessels smooth and wide,
But always monitor the **bleeding tide**.
Clopidogrel—it guards the flow,
But nurses guide how far to go.
With smart checks and bleeding scan,
You'll help this med do all it can.

ENALAPRIL (VASOTEC)
Antihypertensive - ACE Inhibitor

Enalapril—an **ACE** that rules,
It **blocks the enzyme** breaking the fuel.
No **angiotensin II** is made,
So **vasoconstriction** starts to fade.
Used in **hypertension** first,
And **heart failure** when hearts are cursed.
Also helps with **diabetic kidneys**,
Slows down damage, clears the giddies.

It drops the **BP**, calms the heart,
But nurses play a key, smart part.
Side effects? Be on patrol—
Dry cough that takes a stubborn toll.
Also risk for **hyperkalemia**,
So skip **K+ rich diets**, anemia.
And **angioedema** is a fear—
Swollen lips or tongue? Get help near.

Monitor BP and **K+ labs**,
And kidney function with your tabs.
BUN, creatinine may rise,
So follow values, not just eyes.
Teach patients to **rise up slow**,
Orthostatic drops may show.
And warn: **No salt substitutes**,
They're full of **potassium loot**.

It **interacts** with **NSAIDs**, too,
Which blunt its strength and pressure view.
Also **diuretics** raise the risk,
Of **hypotension**—don't be brisk.
No Black Box Warning, but still heed—
Pregnancy? Then stop the feed.
It's **fetal toxic**, not okay,
Especially after the first-trimester day.

Enalapril—a helpful start,
When pressure's high or fails the heart.
With **labs, vitals**, and knowledge bright,
This ACE helps patients sleep at night.

64

ENOXAPARIN (LOVENOX)
Anticoagulant – Low Molecular Weight Heparin (LMWH)

Enoxaparin keeps clots away,
A **low-weight heparin** used each day.
It stops **factor Xa** in the line,
So **DVTs** and **PEs** decline.
Used for **clot prevention** post-surgery,
Or to treat **active clots** with urgency.
Also given for **unstable angina**,
And **MI** in the early arena.
It's given **subQ**—not IV or oral,
With **love handles** as the injection portal.
Never expel the **air bubble inside**,
It helps the **dose stay just right** and glide.
Side effects include **bleeding risk**,
So monitor signs that show up brisk:
Bruising, black stools, hematuria,
And sudden **drop in hemoglobinia**.

Rare but real is **HIT in view**—
That's **heparin-induced thrombocytopenia** too.
Check **platelets** every day,
If they drop fast—stop right away.
Monitor CBC, H&H,
But **aPTT** is not the path.
Unlike heparin, you **don't need routine labs**,
But keep watch close with bleeding tabs.
Black Box Warning you must cite:
Spinal/epidural hematoma fright.
If patient's had a **spinal tap** or block,
Use with caution—**bleeds may knock**.

Teach them **not to rub the site**,
And to rotate spots left and right.
No **NSAIDs** or **aspirin games**,
Unless prescriber clearly names.
Antidote? That's **protamine**,
But it works less well than in heparin's scene.
So **prevention first**, be smart and wise—
Keep bleeding risk from a surprise.
Enoxaparin—a clot's decline,
But nursing care must align.
With teaching, labs, and eyes that see,
You'll guard your patient carefully.

EPTIFIBATIDE (INTEGRILIN)
Antiplatelet - Glycoprotein IIb/IIIa Inhibitor

Eptifibatide, a platelet block,
It halts the **final clotting lock**.
It binds to **GPIIb/IIIa**,
To **stop aggregation** right away.
Used for **unstable angina** pain,
Or **NSTEMI** with cardiac strain.
Also used in **PCI**,
To keep the stent and vessel free.

It's given **IV**, with dosing weight-based,
And often with **heparin** interlaced.
It works real fast—but short it stays,
So keep the **drip** on through the days.
Side effects? **Bleeding risk** is key—
From **gums, urine**, or **GI** spree.
Thrombocytopenia is rare but real,
So check those **platelet labs** with zeal.

Monitor CBC, H&H,
And **aPTT** if heparin's in play.
Watch for **hematuria, bruising**, red,
And hold pressure long where blood was shed.
Don't use in **stroke**, or **bleeding past**,
Or if **thrombocytopenia's** been cast.
Surgery recent? Then don't begin—
The bleeding risk may do them in.

No Black Box Warning, but don't relax,
Renal impairment slows its tracks.
Dose adjust when kidneys stall,
To prevent excess rise and fall.
Teach the team: **No invasive tools**,
Like **NG tubes**, unless by rules.
And **report signs of bleeding fast**,
This antiplatelet's built to last.

Eptifibatide—a clot's delay,
To keep the heart attack at bay.
With **labs and lines**, and nurse's mind,
It's life-saving, used in kind.

HEPARIN
Anticoagulant - Indirect Thrombin Inhibitor

Heparin, fast and powerful flow,
Prevents the **clot** before it can grow.
It binds with **antithrombin III**,
To block **thrombin** and **factor Xa** with glee.
Used for **DVTs**, **PEs**, and more,
MI, **stroke**, and **surgical war**.
It **prevents clots**, not breaks them down,
But keeps new **thrombi** from coming 'round.
Given **IV** or **subQ** with care,
Rapid onset, so nurses beware.
In **drips**, it's **weight-based**, titrated tight,
With labs to guide you left and right.
Side effects? Start with **bleed**,
From gums, urine, or wound that's freed.
Bruising, **hematuria**, **drop in H&H**,
And sudden **back pain** may show a crack.

Watch for **HIT**—a danger deep:
Heparin-induced thrombocytopenia sweep.
Platelets fall, yet clots may form—
A paradoxical, deadly storm.
Monitor aPTT—keep in range,
About **60–80 seconds**, don't let it change.
Check **platelets**, too, and **H&H**,
And signs of **bleeding** you can see.

Black Box Warning must be known:
Spinal hematomas when spine is shown.
Like with **epidurals** or **spinal taps**,
Heparin may cause **permanent relapse**.
Protamine sulfate is the fix,
The **antidote** for bleeding mix.
Given slow through **IV line**,
To reverse the drip and hold the line.
Teach patients: **No aspirin** without say,
And report **bleeding signs** right away.
Soft toothbrush, no razors, please—
Reduce the risks and keep the peace.
Heparin—a high-risk med to lead,
But life-saving when patients bleed.
With **labs**, **teaching**, and eyes on cue,
This drug does what it's meant to do.

IDARUCIZUMAB (PRAXBIND)

Antidote - Direct Reversal Agent for Dabigatran (Pradaxa)

When **dabigatran** leads to a dangerous bleed, **Idarucizumab** is what you'll need. A **monoclonal antibody**, made just right, It grabs the drug and stops the fight.

It's **high-affinity**, fast to bind, Reverses effects in record time. Think trauma, stroke, or urgent knife— This med can **literally save a life**.

It's given **IV**, in two short pushes, And clotting comes back in rapid rushes. Within **minutes**, the work is done— The bleeding slows, the danger's gone.

It's **only for dabigatran**, make that clear, Won't work for apixaban, not even near. If the patient took **Pradaxa**—great, But if not, don't initiate.

No renal dosing adjustments are due, And it's cleared fast once it's through. **No routine labs** are needed to trend— But watch for bleeding until the end.

Don't give it with **heparin** or warfarin's mix, It won't reverse those anticoag tricks. And once you reverse, start planning anew— When to restart their blood thinner too.

It may cause **hypokalemia**, or a **fever**, Some get **delirium**, or chills that shiver. But serious side effects are rare to find— Most reverse safely and do just fine.

If they're getting surgery or brain CT, Make sure this med is ordered quickly. The window to act is narrow and real— You want full reversal before you seal.

Cardiac patients are often the case, With Pradaxa in their pillbox place. So know this name and keep it in mind, For patients bleeding or racing time.

So if dabigatran led to fear, Call for **Praxbind** and get it near. **Idarucizumab** clears the path, And brings them back from Pradaxa's wrath.

PROTAMINE SULFATE
Antidote - Heparin & LMWH Reversal Agent

Protamine Sulfate, the antidote,
For when **heparin's** dose runs afloat.
It binds the med and stops the bleed,
A **reversal agent**—urgent need.
Used in **surgery**, or **bleeding crises**,
When **heparin** causes clotting slices.
Also helps with **enoxaparin**,
Though **partial reversal**—not as darin'.

It's given **IV**, **slow and clear**,
Over **10 minutes**, nurse stays near.
If pushed too fast, don't be shocked—
Hypotension or **brady** gets clocked.
Dose is based on heparin used,
So calculate right—don't be confused.
1 mg of protamine cancels tight,
About **100 units** of heparin's might.

Side effects? Let's list a few:
Flushing, **nausea**, and **hypo** in view.
Watch for **back pain**, **dyspnea**, too,
And allergic response may come through.
Black Box Warning not assigned,
But still, this med needs nurse-aligned.
High risk for **anaphylaxis** dread—
Especially in **fish allergy** or **vasectomy** spread.

So **monitor closely** when it's begun,
Keep **epi** and **O₂** ready to run.
Vitals every **15 minutes**, check,
And stop if signs of shock reflect.
Teach the team: it's not for clots—
It just **neutralizes** what heparin brought.
And if no heparin's in the mix?
Protamine alone can **mess up the fix**.

Protamine Sulfate—antidote elite,
But never one you push on repeat.
With nurse precision and steady hand,
You'll guide reversal as it's planned.

RETEPLASE (RETAVASE)
Thrombolytic - Recombinant Tissue Plasminogen Activator (tPA)

Reteplase, a **clot-busting name**,
Dissolves the **thrombus** fueling the flame.
A **recombinant tPA** drug of choice,
That helps the blocked heart find its voice.
Used in **acute MI**—timing tight,
To restore **perfusion** and save the fight.
Must be given **within 6 hours**,
To stop the damage and restore powers.
It turns on **plasminogen's** role,
To break down **fibrin** and clear the goal.
This cascade melts the clot away,
But bleeding risk comes into play.
Given **IV bolus**, not a drip,
Two doses **30 minutes** apart—quick tip.
Not for stroke or PE use—
That's **alteplase** in that cruise.
Absolute contraindications shout:
Recent **surgery**, **GI bleed**, or clot-out.
Hemorrhagic stroke in history line?
This drug could cross a deadly sign.
Side effects—start with **bleeds**:
From gums, nose, wounds, or surgical deeds.
Also risk of **reperfusion pain**,
Like **arrhythmias** when flow returns again.
Monitor for **hematuria, bruising, ooze**,
And vital signs that start to lose.

Neuro checks should lead your way,
To spot **ICH** without delay.
No Black Box Warning, but high-alert med,
Needs **2 RN checks** before it's fed.
Keep **emergency gear** at side,
And **avoid invasive lines** while it's applied.
Teach the team: it's clot's defeat,
But not without a cautious seat.
And if given with **heparin**, too,
Double-check all labs in view.
Reteplase—fast, aggressive blow,
For **MIs** where time must flow.
With **protocols**, skill, and nurse control,
You'll guide this med to meet its goal.

TENECTEPLASE (TNKASE)

Thrombolytic – Recombinant tPA (Tissue Plasminogen Activator)

Tenecteplase, or **TNKase** short,
Is clot destruction's final resort.
A **recombinant tPA** with flair,
To **lyse the thrombus** then and there.
Used in **STEMI**—MI that's fresh,
It breaks up clots and restores flesh.
IV bolus, one big shot,
Unlike alteplase, which takes a lot.
It **activates plasminogen** fast,
So **fibrin clots** won't long last.
It **melts the clot** to save the heart,
But bleeding risk must play its part.
Absolute contraindications bold:
Active bleeding, **stroke of old**,
Aneurysm, **brain tumors**, **surgery recent**,
Severe hypertension—don't be lenient.
Side effects you'll surely track:
Intracranial hemorrhage leads the pack.
Also **GI bleeds**, **bruising**, and more,
So vitals and **neuro checks** galore.
Check for **reperfusion pain** as well—
It may cause **arrhythmias** to swell.
PVCs, **VT**, even **A-fib**,
As oxygen floods the dying fib.
No Black Box Warning, but this is high-alert,
With **two RN checks** to avoid the hurt.
Once it's given, **no pokes or sticks**,
Avoid invasive lines or tricks.
Must be used within the **3 to 6 hour span**,
From symptom start—that's the plan.
Paired with **heparin** and **aspirin**, too,
Unless bleeding risk is breaking through.
Teach your team: it's not for stroke—
Just **MI**—that's the focus spoke.
One push dose, then monitor tight,
To keep that patient in the light.
Tenecteplase—a thrombus foe,
To get that **ischemic heart** to go.
With **timing**, **labs**, and nurse command,
You'll guide this med with steady hand.

TICAGRELOR (BRILINTA)
Antiplatelet - P2Y12 Inhibitor

Ticagrelor, a platelet block,
Keeps those clots from forming shock.
A **P2Y12 receptor foe**,
It stops the **platelet plug** from flow.
Used in **ACS**, **MI's wrath**,
And **stents** to keep a clearer path.
Often paired with **aspirin low**,
For **dual antiplatelet** power show.
Oral med, with **twice a day** dose,
But **adherence** must be close.
It's not a **blood thinner** per se,
But stops platelets from joining the fray.
Side effects? Let's list a few:
Bleeding risk is front and true.
Epistaxis, **bruises**, **GI bleeds**,
Even **brain bleeds** in rare leads.

Also may cause **dyspnea** mild,
A common quirk, especially wild.
But if **severe**, report it fast—
Breathing struggles should not last.
Black Box Warning—hear this clear:
Don't take with **high-dose aspirin** near.
Over **100 mg daily** may
Reduce this med's protective sway.
So stick to **baby aspirin** style,
Unless the doc adjusts your file.
And **stop 5 days before surgery**,
To lower bleeding risk surgically.

Monitor for signs of stroke or bleed,
Neuro checks, **stools**, and all you need.
Avoid in those with **active bleeds**,
Or **liver disease** that strongly impedes.
Teach: Take it **same time** every day,
And don't **miss doses** or drift away.
Tell your dentist or surgeon crew,
That you're on Brilinta—safety, too.
Ticagrelor—a clot's defeat,
But only safe with a nurse on beat.
With **labs**, **teaching**, and signs reviewed,
You'll guide this med with skill imbued.

TIROFIBAN (AGGRASTAT)
Antiplatelet - Glycoprotein IIb/IIIa Inhibitor

Tirofiban, the platelet block,
Works when clots are set to shock.
A **GP IIb/IIIa inhibitor**, strong,
It stops the platelets from tagging along.
Used in **acute coronary syndrome** flair,
Unstable angina, **MI** care.
Also used in **PCI**,
To keep the arteries clean and high.
IV infusion, titrated slow,
With **bolus dose** to start the flow.
It works by blocking the final path,
Where **platelet cross-linking** sparks its wrath.
Side effects? You know the deal:
Bleeding risk from head to heel.
GI bleeds, **hematuria**, **ooze**,
And rare **intracranial** ones to peruse.

No Black Box Warning, but handle wise—
This med needs **constant nurse eyes**.
Monitor **platelets**, **Hgb**, **Hct**,
And signs of **active bleeds** on the spot.
Contraindications you must know:
Active bleeding, **surgery**, **stroke** in tow.
Also **aneurysm**, **retinal bleed**,
Or **thrombocytopenia** in the lead.
Check for **bradycardia**, **hypotension** drop,
And **monitor ECG** non-stop.
May cause **thrombocytopenia** fast,
So hold the med if platelets don't last.

Given with **heparin** and **aspirin** oft,
To keep that clotting cascade soft.
But with triple therapy comes risk—
So bleeding checks must be brisk.
Teach your team: it's not for home,
Only **in-patient**, ICU zone.
And **stop before surgery**, hours due,
Per **protocol**—not just what feels true.
Tirofiban—a platelet gate,
To stop the clots before it's too late.
With **vigilance**, **labs**, and ICU grace,
You'll run this drip in the safest place.

TRANEXAMIC ACID (CYKLOKAPRON)
Antifibrinolytic - Hemostatic Agent

Tranexamic Acid, clot's best friend,
Helps the **bleeding episode** end.
An **antifibrinolytic** hero,
That keeps **clot breakdown** close to zero.
It blocks **plasminogen's** turn to **plasmin**,
So clots stay firm—not collapsing.
Used in **heavy bleeding** of many kinds—
Surgery, trauma, and **OB lines**.
In **postpartum hemorrhage**, it shines bright,
To help the **uterus clamp down tight**.
Also used in **menstrual flood**,
To slow the loss and save the blood.
IV, oral, even **topical**, too—
The route depends on what you do.
In trauma, give it **within 3 hours**,
To stop internal bleeding powers.

Side effects are usually mild:
Nausea, cramps, maybe **vision riled**.
But rarely, clots may go too bold—
DVT, PE, or **stroke** unfold.
No Black Box Warning, but use with care
In patients with **clot history** to spare.
Retinal occlusion may occur,
So eye symptoms? Check for blur.
Avoid in those with **active clot**,
Or **hematuria** that hits the spot
From **upper tract**, where clot might stay—
And cause obstruction along the way.
Teach: Take with or just after food,
To ease the **GI** attitude.
And not for those on **hormone pills**,
Unless cleared—due to clotting thrills.
Check **CBC, creatinine,** too,
In renal patients passing through.
And always ask about their past—
If they've had **thrombosis**, you must ask.
Tranexamic Acid—a clot's strong shield,
For when the bleeding must be sealed.
With **timing, labs,** and nursing might,
You'll guard each drop with practiced sight.

WARFARIN (COUMADIN)
Anticoagulant - Vitamin K Antagonist

Warfarin, the clot delay,
Keeps **thrombosis** far at bay.
A **vitamin K antagonist**, true,
It blocks the **clotting factors** coming through.
Used for **DVT**, **PE**, and **stroke prevent**,
For **A-fib**, and valve replacement event.
Keeps blood flowing, thin and neat,
But needs **INR checks** to stay on beat.

Goal INR is usually **2 to 3**,
Or **2.5 to 3.5** with valve history.
Too low? You risk another clot.
Too high? A **bleeding** risk is what you've got.
Side effects include **bleeding bright**—
Black stools, bruising, gums that fight.
Nosebleeds, headache, sudden pain,
Could mean a **hemorrhage** in the brain.

Black Box Warning: Bleeds can be fatal,
So monitor labs and keep things stable.
Teach: No **NSAIDs**, or **aspirin**, too,
Unless the doc says it's safe to do.
Vitamin K is the **antidote**,
For bleeding risk or overdose.
So go easy on the **greens you eat**,
But **keep intake steady**—don't cheat or repeat.

Takes several days for effect to rise,
So a **heparin bridge** might be wise.
And never stop it all at once—
Clot risk climbs with such a stunt.
Teach to take it **same time daily**,
And **wear a med alert**—not just maybe.
Report **falls, bleeds**, or **headache sharp**,
And keep your **INR in the chart**.

Warfarin—a clot's dela
But only safe the **nursing way**.
With **labs, education**, and a steady hand,
You'll guide this med as nurses planned.

Part IV
Neurologic & Seizure Management

DANTROLENE (DANTRIUM)

Skeletal Muscle Relaxant - Direct-Acting

Dantrolene calms the muscles' fire,
When **rigid spasms** build up higher.
It works **directly on the muscle site**,
Blocking **calcium release** from flight.
It's the **antidote for malignant heat**,
Malignant hyperthermia can't compete.
Also used for **spastic states**,
Like **MS**, **CP**, or trauma fates.

Side effects? They can appear:
Drowsiness, dizziness, weakness near.
May cause **GI upset**, too,
Like **nausea, diarrhea** in view.
But nurses, here's a vital tip:
Watch out for **liver toxicity slip**.
Check **AST, ALT**, with care—
Hepatotoxicity can flare.

There's a **Black Box Warning** on the sheet:
For **liver failure**, rare but deep.
Especially in **females over 35**,
Monitor labs to keep them alive.
Teach: Avoid **alcohol** and **CNS depressants**,
That makes sedation more unpleasant.
Report **jaundice, fatigue**, or pain,
In **upper right quadrant**—don't let it remain.

For **IV use**, it's given fast,
In OR rooms where temps rise fast.
Dilute and mix it **right before**,
Stability fades—it won't last more.
Used with **anesthesia**? Yes, indeed—
To stop that **hypermetabolic speed**.
It **relaxes muscles**, cools the core,
So patients can return to norm once more.

Dantrolene—a muscle's peace,
But nurse, beware before release.
With sharp eyes and patient cues,
You'll help them walk in steadier shoes.

FOSPHENYTOIN (CEREBYX)

Fosphenytoin, a prodrug start,
Converts to **phenytoin** to do its part.
Used to stop a **seizure storm**,
And keep the brain **electrically warm**.
Treats **status epilepticus** fast,
And helps with seizures that always last.
Also used for **seizure prevention**
After **neurosurgery** or brain tension.
Given **IV or IM** with care,
It's **less caustic** than phenytoin's flare.
No **purple glove syndrome** risk in play—
It's safer when you need to act today.
Side effects? You'll still need eyes:
Bradycardia, **hypotension**, might arise.
Also **dizziness**, **nystagmus**, **rash**,
Or **CNS depression** in a flash.

Monitor **BP**, **EKG**, and rate,
And check for **toxicity** before it's too late.
Look for signs like **ataxia**, **slurred speech**,
Or **confusion** just out of reach.
It's dosed in **PEs** (phenytoin equivalents),
So check the math with **ordered measurements**.

And **infuse slow**—don't let it rush,
Too fast may cause a cardiac crush.
No Black Box Warning, but don't forget:
It still can cause **Steven-Johnson threat**,
Especially in those with **Asian descent**,
So **genetic testing** may be sent.
Drug interactions? Yes, a lot—
It's a **CYP inducer** in the drug pot.
Can lower levels of many meds,
From **warfarin** to **oral contraceptive threads**.
Teach patients if switching to oral pill,
That **phenytoin levels** must be stable still.
And teach about **oral hygiene game**—
To prevent **gingival overgrowth** by name.
Fosphenytoin—smooth and fast,
For seizure care that's built to last.
With **vitals**, **labs**, and nurse command,
You'll dose this med with expert hand.

LACOSAMIDE (VIMPAT)
Anticonvulsant - Sodium Channel Enhancer

When **partial seizures** spark and flare, And other drugs don't get them there, **Lacosamide** steps in with grace— To help slow down the firing pace.

It works by **enhancing sodium gates**, Stabilizing neurons before it's too late. It keeps them calm and less excitable, So seizure spread is less reliable.

It's used in **focal seizures**, both new and old, And sometimes in **status**, when things unfold. Given **oral or IV**, with titration slow, Start low, go slow, and let the dose grow.

Dizziness and **diplopia** top the list, Of side effects you won't want to miss. **Nausea, fatigue,** or **vertigo** too— So monitor closely when starting anew.

It may **prolong PR** on an EKG, So get a baseline and trend what you see. **Caution in cardiac** patients is wise, Especially if conduction issues arise.

Don't stop suddenly—**seizure rebound** is real, Wean it down slow, that's part of the deal. And if they're already prone to depression, Watch mood and thoughts with clear expression.

Suicidal ideation has been reported, So mental health checks should be supported. Report signs of **confusion**, withdrawal, or tears, Especially in the early weeks or years.

Tell patients not to drive right away— Until they know how they feel each day. **Fall risk rises** with blurry sight, And dizziness might strike at night.

Interactions? Not too bad— But **CNS depressants** can make things sad. So careful with benzos, opioids, and wine— Too much can cross a dangerous line.

Monitor **labs** for **LFT elevation**, Especially in those with known liver limitation. And though it's rare, a **rash** could show— Call the provider if symptoms grow.

For focal seizures with stubborn streak, **Lacosamide** may be the tweak you seek. Just dose it slow and monitor wise, To keep their brain from seizing surprise.

LEVETIRACETAM (KEPPRA)

Anticonvulsant

Keppra helps the brain when seizures strike,
It keeps things calm when sparks don't act right.
Used for **partial, tonic-clonic,** or **general** type,
It controls the storm when neurons hype.
Though the **exact mechanism's** not crystal clear,
It modulates **neurotransmitters**—keeps firing in gear.
No need for levels like with **phenytoin**,
And **fewer interactions**, so patients join in.

It can cause **drowsiness, fatigue, dizzy spells**,
And **behavioral changes**—mood that swells.
Watch out for **depression**, or sudden **rage**,
Especially in kids or adolescent age.
Sometimes **Stevens-Johnson** is a rare but feared call,
So **report rashes** or fever, no matter how small.
It's usually well-tolerated—once or twice daily,
IV or **oral**, prescribed quite freely.

Teach not to stop it **abruptly**, beware—
Seizures may worsen and catch unaware.
Encourage good **sleep**, and staying on track,
Missing a dose can bring symptoms back.
For **status epilepticus**, it might be used too,
Alongside **benzos** in that rescue crew.
Pregnancy-safe? It may be okay,
But weigh all the risks in a thoughtful way.

So **Levetiracetam**, steady and smart,
Keeps seizures at bay, does its neuro part.
Well-loved for its ease, and low side effect rates,
A staple med that often rates great.

NALMEFENE

Opioid Antagonist - Antidote for Opioid Overdose

Nalmefene, a rescue call,
Blocks the **opioids** that try to stall.
A **pure antagonist**, strong and clear,
To bring back breath and fight the fear.
It binds to **mu, kappa, delta** tight,
And kicks the **opioids** off that site.
Used for **opioid overdose** relief,
Or to reverse **respiratory grief**.

Longer-lasting than **naloxone** is,
So it helps when relapse is the biz.
Its **half-life** stays a little more,
To block the **rebound sedation** score.
Given **IV, IM**, or **subQ**,
Onset's fast—**within minutes, too**.
But dose with care and **watch the vibe**,
It can **trigger withdrawal** that's hard to ride.

Side effects to monitor near:
Hypertension, agitation, sweating fear.
Also **nausea, vomiting**, pain returns,
As **opioid blocks** make cravings burn.
Tachycardia, seizures, can arise,
Especially in patients who've used high.
So **monitor vitals, O₂ sat**, and more,
And keep **airway support** at the door.

No Black Box Warning yet assigned,
But treat like **naloxone**—stay aligned.
In overdose cases, stay alert,
As **Nalmefene** can still **uncover hurt**.
Teach the team: It's **not a cure**,
But a **bridge to breathing**, safe and sure.
Always call for **911**,
Even when reversal's done.

Nalmefene—a longer guard,
To keep **opioid OD** from hitting hard.
With **monitoring**, prep, and nurse-led grace,
You'll keep your patient in a safe place.

NALOXONE (NARCAN)
Opioid Antagonist - Antidote for Opioid Overdose

Naloxone, fast and lifesaving name,
Reverses **opioids** in their game.
It binds to **mu receptors** tight,
And kicks out **morphine, fentanyl, Dilaudid**—right.
Used for **opioid overdose** events,
With **respiratory depression** as the defense.
Also used post-surgery scene,
To reverse **sedation** that gets too keen.

Can be given **IV, IM, subQ**, or **nasal spray**,
And works within **1–2 minutes**—no delay.
But its **half-life** is often short,
So **repeat dosing** may need support.
Side effects come fast and strong,
Like **withdrawal symptoms** all day long:
Agitation, vomiting, tachycardia kick,
Sweating, pain, and **nausea quick.**

If dependent, they may shout or cry,
Because Narcan makes the **high goodbye**.
So always watch with gentle grace—
You're saving lives, not judging face.
No Black Box Warning, but beware:
The risk of **rebound overdose** is there.

As opioids may **outlast Narcan's aid**,
So keep close watch as vitals fade.

Monitor **respiratory rate and depth**,
Check **O₂ saturation** with each breath.
Have **resuscitation gear** nearby,
Because the crash can come back by.
Teach: Call **911**, don't walk away,
Even if they seem **okay**.
And train families how to spray—
So they're prepared to save the day.

Naloxone (Narcan)—a life restart,
The breath that wakes a silent heart.
With **timing, skill**, and nursing might,
You'll bring them safely back to light.

84

NEOSTIGMINE
Cholinergic - Acetylcholinesterase Inhibitor

Neostigmine, sharp and true,
Boosts **acetylcholine** to push it through.
An **acetylcholinesterase inhibitor**,
That makes nerve signals **stronger and quicker**.
Used in **myasthenia gravis** flares,
To help restore the **strength impaired**.
Also used to **reverse** the scene,
Of **neuromuscular block** post-surgery clean.
It keeps **acetylcholine** around,
So **muscles move** with strength unbound.
Given **IV**, **IM**, or sometimes oral,
Its timing needs to be quite formal.
Side effects are often wet:
Salivation, **nausea**, **sweating** set.
Also **bradycardia**, **cramps**, and **pee**,
The classic **SLUDGE** signs you'll see:
**Salivation, Lacrimation, Urination,
Diarrhea, GI upset, Emesis**—full activation.
Risk of **cholinergic crisis** grows,
If too much neostigmine flows.
So distinguish from **myasthenic crash**—
That's when the dose may need a dash.
No Black Box Warning, but take care—
Respiratory failure could be there.
If muscles of **breathing** get too weak,
They'll need support before they speak.

Antidote? Yes! It's **atropine**,
To reverse the **cholinergic** machine.
Keep it close if you go high,
And monitor vitals by and by.
Check for **improved strength**, chewing right,
Less drooping eyes and **breathing tight**.
But dose it same time every day,
To keep the weakness far away.

Neostigmine—a steady hand,
To help the nerves and muscles stand.
With careful checks and nurse finesse,
You'll guide each dose to patient success.

85

PHENYTOIN (DILANTIN)
Anticonvulsant - Sodium Channel Blocker

Phenytoin, steady and slow,
Keeps the **neurons** from overflow.
It blocks those **sodium channels** tight,
To stop the sparks from taking flight.
Used for **seizures**—tonic-clonic bold,
And **status epilepticus** when uncontrolled.
Also may prevent post-surgery flare,
In **neurosurgery** ICU care
Given **oral** or by **IV route**,
But give it slow—**watch out! watch out!**
IV push too fast can **tank BP**,
Or cause **arrhythmias** suddenly.
Side effects? A list to learn:
Gingival hyperplasia—watch the turn.
Hirsutism, rash, and **CNS haze**,
Like **drowsy, ataxia, vision daze**.
Can cause **Stevens-Johnson Syndrome**, too,
A **skin reaction** rare but true.
And long-term use may cause decline
In **vitamin D** and **folic line**.
Black Box Warning to address:
For **cardiovascular risk** with IV stress.
Too fast a push can make things slip,
So always use **on a pump** or **drip**
Monitor **levels**—they're narrow in range:
10 to 20 mcg/mL is the exchange.

Too low? Seizures may still stay.
Too high? Toxic side effects all day.
Toxicity signs you need to know:
Nystagmus, slurred speech, gait that's slow.
If those show up, check the chart,
You may be dosing off the mark.
Interacts with many meds—
It's an **enzyme inducer**, not just heads.
So **warfarin, birth control**, may change,
And other drug levels rearrange.
Teach to take at the **same time each day**,
Don't **stop abruptly** or seizures may play.
Good **oral hygiene** is a must,
Or **gum overgrowth** breaks the trust.
Phenytoin—a seizure guide,
But only safe with nurse beside.
With **labs, vitals**, and a watchful plan,
You'll guide this med like only a nurse can.

PHENOBARBITAL
Barbiturate - Anticonvulsant / Sedative-Hypnotic

Phenobarbital, old but strong,
Keeps **seizures** from staying long.
A **barbiturate** with **GABA flair**,
It calms the brain and clears the air.
Used for **tonic-clonic seizures** loud,
And **febrile seizures** in the child crowd.
Also helps with **status epilepticus**,
When newer meds just don't assist.
It **enhances GABA**—a calming key,
To slow **neuronal activity**.
Given **oral**, **IM**, or **IV fast**,
Its **sedation effects** can last and last.
Side effects? They come with weight:
Drowsiness, lethargy, slowed-up state.
Depression, ataxia, mood decline,
And **respiratory depression** is the sign.

Black Box Warning to be told:
Abuse potential—strong and bold.
Dependence, tolerance, and **withdrawal pain**—
Taper slow or risk the strain.
Monitor **RR**, **LOC**, and tone,
Especially when given **IV alone**.
Watch for **hypotension, bradycardia**, too,
And **toxicity signs** that come into view.
Check **levels**—it has a **narrow range**,
And too much can quickly rearrange.
Therapeutic window is 15-40,
Above that line, it's not too sporty.

Enzyme inducer—yep, it speeds
The breakdown of **other meds** and leads
To lowered drug levels, less effect—
So med interactions must be checked.
Teach to take it the **same time daily**,
And avoid stopping **suddenly or gaily**.
Driving? Only when stable and clear,
And no **alcohol** or CNS depressants near.
Phenobarbital—an older friend,
With seizure-blocking power to lend.
But used with care, and steady track,
To keep the CNS on the right track.

PROPAFENONE (RYTHMOL)

Antiarrhythmic - Class Ic Sodium Channel Blocker

Propafenone, heart rhythm's guide,
A **Class Ic** drug that modifies the ride.
It blocks the **sodium channels** strong,
To slow **conduction** when rhythms go wrong.
Used for **atrial fibrillation** to convert,
Atrial flutter, **PSVT**, and prevent the hurt.
Also treats some **ventricular beats**,
But only in hearts without **structural defeats**.

Oral med, with a narrow path,
Must monitor well to avoid wrath.
Has some **beta-blocker** flair inside,
So **slows the rate** with rhythm tied.
Side effects you must surveil:
Bradycardia, **hypotension**, pale.
Dizziness, **fatigue**, or bitter taste,
And **bronchospasm**—so **asthmatics**? Waste.

Black Box Warning stands so bold:
Proarrhythmic risk in hearts not whole.
In **post-MI**, or **structural strain**,
It may cause **VT**, **VF**, or pain.
Can widen the **QRS** or **PR**,
So monitor with **EKG on par**.
Check **liver**, **renal**, and **drug level flow**,
And **hold the dose** if rhythms go.

It interacts with many meds,
Like **digoxin**, **warfarin**—watch your threads.
It raises levels, slows the pace,
So dose adjustments fall in place.
Teach: Take the pill the **same time daily**,
No skipping or stopping gaily.
And if they feel **palpitations** rise,
Report it fast—don't compromise.

Propafenone—a potent thread,
To guide the beat and clear the dread.
But only used with nurse finesse,
To keep the rhythm calm and less.

VALPROIC ACID (DEPAKOTE)

Anticonvulsant / Mood Stabilizer

Valproic Acid, steady and strong,
Keeps the **neurons** from firing wrong.
It boosts **GABA**, calms the brain,
And quiets down **epileptic strain**.
Used for **seizures**, **bipolar** highs,
And **migraine prevention**—quite the prize.
A go-to **mood stabilizer** tool,
Especially when **mania** breaks the rule.
It blocks **sodium channels** wide,
So **neuronal firing** can subside.
But it's not without its flags—
So nurses, watch for warning tags.
Side effects? They top the charts:
Tremor, **weight gain**, **hair that parts**.
Also **GI upset**, **drowsy tone**,
And **thrombocytopenia** shown.
Black Box Warnings—there are three:
- **Hepatotoxicity**, especially early.
- **Pancreatitis**, rare but grim, With **abdominal pain** and danger dim.
- And **teratogenic risks**—severe, In pregnancy, it's nowhere near.

Causes **neural tube defects**,
So use in childbearing age? Complex.
Teach to use **reliable birth control**,
And discuss the risks in full control.
Monitor **LFTs**, and **amylase**, too,
And **platelets**, since bleeding could ensue.

Check **drug levels** to stay in range—
50 to 100 is not too strange.
Can interact with other meds,
So check the list before it spreads.
Increases levels of **phenobarb** and more,
And **lamotrigine rash** could soar.
Teach: Take with food if stomach turns,
And watch for **yellow skin that burns**.
Report **bruising, bleeding, mood shifts** fast,
And **don't stop suddenly**—seizures blast.
Valproic Acid—brain's control,
But only safe with nurse patrol.
With **labs, education**, and patient trust,
You'll guide this med with skills robust.

89

Part V
Reversal Agents & Toxicology

ACETYLCYSTEINE (MUCOMYST)

Mucolytic / Antidote

Acetylcysteine, a helper true,
Does more than most of us ever knew.
A **mucolytic**, it thins the goo,
And serves as an **antidote** too.
It **breaks disulfide bonds** with ease,
So **thick mucus** turns to flowing seas.
In lungs, it makes the airways clear—
For **COPD**, it's held quite dear.

But if **Tylenol** takes a toll,
And **liver failure** is the goal,
This drug steps in to **replenish GSH**—
Protects the liver in a dash.
Use it for:
Acetaminophen overdose,
Chronic bronchitis, mucus gross.
Contrast nephropathy prevention too,
It's versatile—yes, that's true!

Watch for **nausea**, **vomit**, **rash**, and more,
A **bronchospasm** may be in store.
It smells like **rotten eggs**, beware,
So give a heads-up—show you care.
Nurses, prep it right away,
If it's oral, mix it—mask the taste, okay?
In IV form, check **renal labs**,
Liver enzymes, don't let it lapse.

Administer within 8-10 hours
Of overdose—then watch its powers.
Monitor for signs of **anaphylactoid**,
Especially IV—be paranoid.
Teach the patient it may smell,
And **vomit** too, but it works well.
Encourage fluids, cough it out—
Hydration helps to move it out.

Though there's **no black box warning** here,
Reactions still may bring some fear.
Give a **test dose** if they're at risk,
And **slow the rate** if it gets brisk.
Interactions? Not a ton—
But **activated charcoal** can ruin the fun.
It binds and blocks if given too near,
So **space them out** to keep it clear.

Acetylcysteine, with many roles,
From clearing lungs to saving souls.
A nurse's tool, both sharp and kind—
With timing crucial, keep that in mind.

ANDEXANET ALFA
Antidote - Factor Xa Inhibitor Reversal Agent

When **dabigatran** leads to a dangerous bleed, **Idarucizumab** is what you'll need. A **monoclonal antibody**, made just right, It grabs the drug and stops the fight.
It's **high-affinity**, fast to bind, Reverses effects in record time. Think trauma, stroke, or urgent knife— This med can **literally save a life**.
It's given **IV**, in two short pushes, And clotting comes back in rapid rushes. Within **minutes**, the work is done— The bleeding slows, the danger's gone.
It's **only for dabigatran**, make that clear, Won't work for apixaban, not even near. If the patient took **Pradaxa**—great, But if not, don't initiate.
No renal dosing adjustments are due, And it's cleared fast once it's through. **No routine labs** are needed to trend— But watch for bleeding until the end.
Don't give it with **heparin** or warfarin's mix, It won't reverse those anticoag tricks. And once you reverse, start planning anew— When to restart their blood thinner too.
It may cause **hypokalemia**, or a **fever**, Some get **delirium**, or chills that shiver. But serious side effects are rare to find— Most reverse safely and do just fine.
If they're getting surgery or brain CT, Make sure this med is ordered quickly. The window to act is narrow and real— You want full reversal before you seal.
Cardiac patients are often the case, With Pradaxa in their pillbox place. So know this name and keep it in mind, For patients bleeding or racing time.
So if dabigatran led to fear, Call for **Praxbind** and get it near. **Idarucizumab** clears the path, And brings them back from Pradaxa's wrath.

Oops! This is actually the **Idarucizumab** poem again! Let me now give you the **correct Andexanet alfa (Andexxa) poem** with the updated subtitle—right below.

Andexanet Alfa *Antidote - Factor Xa Inhibitor Reversal Agent*
When **rivaroxaban** has gone too far, Or **Eliquis** caused a bleeding scar, **Andexanet Alfa** is what you need— A **reversal agent** for a **Factor Xa bleed**.
It mimics Xa and grabs the drug, So clotting resumes without a tug. A **decoy protein**, lab-designed, To neutralize fast and reassign.
Use it for **life-threatening bleeds**, Like **GI hemorrhage** or surgical needs. Give **IV bolus**, then **infuse on a pump**, Monitor close—this isn't a slump.
It's **only for rivaroxaban or apixaban**— Won't help with Pradaxa or fondaparinux's plan. So verify meds before you begin, Because not all anticoagulants fit in.
Watch for thrombosis after the drip, Clotting rebounds and starts to grip. **MI, stroke**, or **DVT** may rise— So don't relax after bleeding subsides.
No reversal agent is needed for this one— It wears off fast when the drip is done. Just **monitor labs**, assess the bleed, And plan the next step based on need.
Avoid giving with **heparin too**, It binds and blocks it—that won't do. No major food or drug surprise, But it's still new—so supervise.
It's **expensive**, so use with care, And only when things are truly rare. Like a bleed that won't stop, or a CT bleed— Andexxa's the one for that urgent need.
Teach the team to act with speed, And know which med caused the bleed. Because if you guess the wrong one here, The bleed may spread, and outcomes veer.
So when **Xa inhibitors** go off script, And a patient starts to hemorrhage or slip, Call for **Andexxa**, don't delay— It may just save a life that day.

DIGOXIN IMMUNE FAB (DIGIFAB)

Antidote – Digoxin-Specific Antibody Fragments

When **digoxin levels** rise too high, And your patient's heart might say goodbye, **DigiFab** steps in, the rescue made, With **antibody fragments** professionally laid.

It binds to **free digoxin** in the blood, Neutralizing poison before the flood. Then both are cleared through **renal flow**, So kidneys must work for things to go.

Used in **toxicity** that threatens life, Like **bradycardia**, **heart block**, or rhythm strife. Also if **K is high** while dig is strong— That's a combo that won't last long.

You'll see signs like **vision turned green**, **GI distress** or arrhythmias unseen. Nausea, vomiting, confusion, and more— These are red flags you can't ignore.

Draw a **serum dig level** before you treat, But don't wait for labs if the rhythm's beat. Dose is based on **amount ingested**, Or level and weight if it's been tested.

Give IV slowly, and filter the line— Anaphylaxis can happen in time. Keep **crash cart** near and monitor well, Especially if allergies start to swell.

After giving, **don't recheck dig**, Because bound levels still show up big. They'll read as high, though they're inactive— So don't let that lab make things reactive.

Watch potassium—it may fall quick, Once dig's reversed, it drops like a brick. Hypokalemia can cause more arrhythmia, So replace it gently with rhythm criteria.

No routine dosing—this one's rare, So document well and handle with care. Not for mild symptoms or slight confusion, Use only in **true cardiac diffusion**.

It's pregnancy-safe if the need is strong, Better reversal than letting things go wrong. Just teach them why their heart flipped bad— And how **DigiFab** reversed what they had.

So when **digoxin overdose** takes the stage, And rhythm's chaos starts to rage, DigiFab neutralizes the toxic med— To keep the patient safe instead.

FLUMAZENIL (ROMAZICON)

Flumazenil, a reversal key,
For **benzos** like **Valium**, **Ativan**, **Versed**, you see.
It **blocks GABA receptors** on the spot,
So **sedation**, **drowsiness**, starts to stop.
Used for **benzo overdose**, **procedural wake**,
Or when sedation's more than they can take.
It's **IV push**, works **fast and clean**,
But nurses—there's a risk unseen.

Side effects you must expect:
Seizures, especially if **benzo-dependent** or wrecked.
Also **nausea, dizziness, panic state**,
And **agitation** that won't wait.
Check for **history of seizures** true—
This med can **trigger breakthrough** too.
If they've used **benzos long-term wide**,
Be careful—**withdrawal** may coincide.

Monitor **LOC, RR, O₂**,
And **seizure activity**, too.
Have **rescue meds** and **airway gear**,
And watch the patient closely near.
Black Box Warning is in play:
Seizure risk if you reverse the wrong way.

Especially after **head trauma**,
Or **cyclic antidepressant drama**.

It wears off **faster than the benzo** dose,
So **resedation** might come close.
May need to **repeat the dose again**,
To keep them calm and breathing then.
Teach your team: it's **not a fix**,
But a **temporary reversal** in the mix.
It does **not block alcohol** or other drugs,
So don't assume it clears all bugs.

Flumazenil—a rescue med,
But walk on clinical toes instead.
With close watch, caution, and airway plan,
You'll bring them back as best you can.

HYDROXYCOBALAMIN
Vitamin - Vitamin B12 / Antidote for Cyanide Poisoning

Hydroxycobalamin, red and bright,
Restores the blood and brings back light.
It's **vitamin B12**, strong and true,
For patients lacking the **energy glue**.
Used in **B12 deficiency**,
From **pernicious anemia** to **malabsorption spree**.
Also the **antidote** we keep on hand,
For **cyanide poisoning**—emergency land.
It helps form **RBCs**, nerves, and more,
And boosts **DNA** at the cellular core.
In cyanide cases, it binds the threat,
Forming **cyanocobalamin**—a safer bet.
Given **IM**, or **IV slow**,
Depending on how symptoms go.
For **chronic B12**, it's often long-term,
But for **cyanide**, it's fast and firm.

Side effects? A few to track:
Red skin, **urine**, may come back.
Don't be alarmed—it's just the dye,
But always teach the patient why.
Also can cause **itching**, **rash**,
Hypertension may rise in a flash.
Nausea, **headache**, **swelling face**,
So monitor closely, just in case.
No Black Box Warning, but take care—
IV infusion must go there
With **monitoring for BP shifts**,
As pressure sometimes quickly lifts.
Check **B12 levels, H&H**,
And **reticulocytes** for full effect.
In anemia, teach **diet, too**,
Meat, **eggs**, and **dairy** get them through.
Teach to report **tingling, fatigue**,
And **neuro changes**—don't fatigue.
And with cyanide, time is key—
Administer fast, and **monitor vitally**.

Hydroxycobalamin—a vitamin win,
And **toxin shield** when trouble begins.
With knowledge sharp and nursing hands,
You'll use this med just as it stands.

IDARUCIZUMAB (PRAXBIND)

Antidote - Direct Reversal Agent for Dabigatran (Pradaxa)

Idarucizumab (Praxbind)
Idarucizumab is the name,
Praxbind is its claim to fame.
A monoclonal antibody, no doubt,
To reverse dabigatran when bleeding breaks out.

It binds that drug with high affinity,
Stopping its anticoagulant activity.
Used when emergent surgery's planned,
Or uncontrolled bleeds get out of hand.

Administered IV, no time to waste—
Two doses of 2.5 grams, spaced.
Onset's within minutes, fast and wise,
To lower the risk of fatal demise.

Watch for hypokalemia, fever, and chills,
And clot formation—yes, that kills.
Risk for thromboembolic events is real,
Like DVT, PE, or a stroke ordeal.

Check aPTT and signs of a clot,
Like leg pain, swelling, or breathing that's not.
No need to adjust for renal strain,
But still check creatinine just in case of pain.

Teach the patient this isn't a cure,
Just reverses Pradaxa, fast and pure.

Let them know that bleeding might end,
But stroke prevention will still depend.

Avoid use with other anticoags,
Until you reassess and clear the fog.
And document timing—don't delay,
This med works best right away.

There's no black box warning yet to date,
But monitor closely and communicate.
Idarucizumab—short and sweet,
A life-saving reversal that can't be beat

INTRALIPID
IV Fat Emulsion – Parenteral Nutrition / Lipid Rescue Agent

Intralipid, a milky flow,
A **fat emulsion** nurses know.
It fuels the body **when NPO**,
And sometimes saves from **drug overdose**.
Used in **TPN** to meet fat needs,
It provides the **essential lipids** feeds.
Calories, energy, **fat-soluble aids**,
When the gut can't join the feeding parade.

Also used as **lipid rescue**, quick—
For **local anesthetic toxicity** thick.
Like **bupivacaine** that won't wear down,
Intralipid turns the case around.
IV only, hung with care,
Through a **separate line** or filtered air.
Inspect the bag for **clumps or breaks**,
Emulsion separation—don't make mistakes.

Side effects are mostly rare:
Fever, nausea, maybe air.
But watch for signs of **fat overload**,
Like **enlarged liver**, or **platelet road**.
Check **triglycerides** before you start,
Too high a level may harm the heart.
Can also raise **pancreatitis** risk,
So **monitor labs** and don't just whisk.

No Black Box Warning, but don't forget—
Allergy to eggs? A safety threat.
Made from **soybean oil** and **egg yolk**,
So assess before that IV poke.
In **lipid rescue**, it binds the drug,
And pulls it from the heart's tight hug.
So in emergencies, it plays a role—
A **fatty sponge** with a life-saving goal.

Intralipid—for fuel or fight,
With nursing hands, you'll dose it right.
From **nutrition bags** to **code cart flair**,
This milky med needs thoughtful care.

METHYLENE BLUE
Antidote - Methemoglobinemia Reversal Agent

When **oxygen's there** but won't let go, And blood turns dark with a chocolate flow, **Methylene Blue** steps in to say, "Let's bring those red cells back today."

It treats **methemoglobinemia**, rare but real, When iron's in a state that won't help you heal. It shifts **Fe^{3+} back to Fe^{2+}**, so quick, Letting hemoglobin bind oxygen slick.

You'll see it after **nitrate drugs**, Or certain **toxins**, or dapsone bugs. When pulse ox shows low, but PaO_2's fine, That's a clue it's **methemoglobin** time.

Give **IV slowly**, dilute the dose, Watch for **site irritation** the most. Usually a **1-2 mg/kg hit**, Over 5 minutes—it's over quick.

It turns the **urine blue** and **stool may stain**, So warn your patient so they don't complain. **Skin and sclera** may tint a hue, But it fades out fast as it clears through you.

Don't use if the patient has **G6PD deficiency**, It can cause **hemolysis** violently. Check before giving—this point is key, Or you'll swap one crisis for another emergency.

Side effects may be **headache or chest pain**, Or **nausea** if you push it like a train. High doses might bring **serotonin syndrome**, So **watch with SSRIs** or they may foam.

Also used in rare **shock states** too, And as a dye in **surgical view**. But for NCLEX prep and ER charts, It's best known for fixing **chocolate hearts**.

Monitor for return of **pink tone and pulse**, And signs the patient no longer convulse. Check **ABGs** and **O_2 sats rise**, Though pulse ox might still tell some lies.

So if your patient's turning blue, And oxygen's there but won't go through, **Methylene Blue** is your rapid reply— To help the hemoglobin work and oxygen fly.

SODIUM BICARBONATE
Alkalinizing Agent - Electrolyte / Buffer

Sodium Bicarbonate, buffer base,
Restores the **pH** to a safer place.
An **alkalinizing** rescue ride,
When **acidosis** swings too wide.
Used in **metabolic acidosis** sharp,
Or **cardiac arrest** when rhythms harp.
Also helps in **TCA overdose**,
To keep the **QRS** from getting gross.
It **raises serum pH** with care,
By **binding hydrogen ions** in the air.
In **DKA**, or **renal fail**,
It gives the blood a fighting trail.
IV push or **slow infusion**,
But always based on clear conclusion.
Too much can **flip the scale** to high,
Causing **alkalosis** to amplify.

Side effects? Don't let them hide:
Metabolic alkalosis on the other side.
Also **hypokalemia, hypocalcemia** arise—
So watch for **tetany, spasms**, or **cries**.
May cause **fluid overload, sodium climb**,
So **CHF** or **renal patients** need time.
And **CO_2 production** goes up high,
Which may increase **ICP** nearby.
No Black Box Warning, but caution strong—
In **resuscitation**, dosing wrong
Can push the blood too far to base,
And worsen outcomes in that race.
Flush the line if mixing drugs—
It can react and form some slugs.
Especially with **calcium chloride's** kind—
That combo? **Precipitate** you'll find.
Teach: It's not a daily med,
But part of the **code cart** instead.
Used in crises, labs in hand,
To **buy some time**, not cure on stand.
Sodium Bicarb—rescue tide,
For **pH crashes** we can't let slide.
With **labs, caution**, and nurse-led care,
You'll buffer life with skill and flair.

Part VI
Antibiotics & Antimicrobials

AZITHROMYCIN (ZITHROMAX)

Antibiotic - Macrolide

Azithromycin fights with grace,
A **macrolide** that holds its place.
It binds to **ribosomes**, shuts down code,
So **protein synthesis** can't load.
It treats **pneumonia**, **strep**, and more,
STIs, and **ear infections** galore.
Also used for **skin** and **sinus** flair,
A broad-spectrum med with gentle care.

Side effects may **upset the gut**—
Think **nausea**, **cramps**, and **diarrhea** rut.
May also cause **QT prolongation**,
So monitor that heart's vibration.
In rare events, **liver** can react—
So watch for **jaundice**, lab track.
Hearing loss may sometimes show,
Especially when the **dose is high or slow**.

Check **LFTs** and **EKG**,
Especially in those with heart history.
Monitor for signs of **superinfection**—
Like **oral thrush** or **newest infection**.
Teach them: **Take it with or without food**,
But **no antacids** close—those change the mood.
Space **aluminum** and **magnesium**, too,
They block absorption coming through.

No **Black Box Warning**, but still take care—
With cardiac risk, you must beware.
It **interacts** with **warfarin**, too,
Can raise bleed risk—so check INR view.
It's long in half-life, hangs around,
So dosing's short, but impact's sound.
Azithromycin, calm and fast,
Fights the bugs and helps them last.

CEFTRIAXONE (ROCEPHIN)
Antibiotic – Third-Generation Cephalosporin

Ceftriaxone, a **cephalosporin**,
Fights off bugs both sly and foreign.
It **inhibits cell wall synthesis**,
So **bacteria break**—they can't persist.
Used in **pneumonia, UTIs,
Sepsis, meningitis,** and **STIs**.
Great for **Gram-negative** strains galore,
And **surgical prophylaxis**, too—what's more!

Side effects are mostly mild,
But **GI upset** may cramp your child.
Rash, itching, or **yeast infection**,
And rarely **Stevens-Johnson reaction**.
But here's the nurse's greatest heed—
Watch out for **biliary sludge** indeed.
Can raise **LFTs** or **cause gallbladder pain**,
Especially in kids—it's not so plain.

Check for **allergy to penicillins**,
Cross-reactivity is one of the villains.
Anaphylaxis may appear,
So keep **airway** meds and **epinephrine** near.
Give it **deep IM** or **IV slow**,
Dilute it right, and watch it flow.
Reconstitute with care and check—
Calcium mix may cause a wreck.

No Black Box Warning, but still proceed—
With **renal checks** and allergy heed.
Avoid with **calcium IV lines**,
They may **crystalize** and cross the signs.
Educate: Complete the course,
Even if they're better, stay the course.
It's one tough med with proven might,
Ceftriaxone—dosed just right.

CIPROFLOXACIN (CIPRO)
Antibiotic - Fluoroquinolone

Ciprofloxacin, bold and wide,
A **fluoroquinolone** antibiotic guide.
It stops **DNA gyrase** with flair,
So bacteria **can't divide or repair**.
Used for **UTIs**, **GI infection**,
Bone, **skin**, and **respiratory protection**.
Anthrax exposure, **traveler's gut**,
And **STIs**—this med packs a punch, no rut.

But side effects? They make some fuss:
Nausea, diarrhea, not much plus.
Tendon rupture, joint pain, sore—
Especially in **aging patients** more.
Watch for **QT prolongation**, too,
And signs of **C. diff** coming through.
Photosensitivity may flare—
So teach them: **Avoid strong sun glare**.

Monitor for **pain in tendons**,
Especially **Achilles**—don't pretend.
It can also cause **CNS distress**—
Confusion, restlessness, more or less.
Take it **on an empty gut**,
But not with **milk** or **iron**—cut!
Antacids, too, should be spaced far,
They block absorption from this star.

No **Black Box Warning** gets ignored:
Tendinitis and **tendon rupture** scored.
Also risk of **peripheral nerve pain**,
And **mood shifts** that are hard to explain.

Interacts with **warfarin**, **theophylline**, too,
So monitor levels, just to be true.
Hydration's key—keep **urine flowing**,
To keep those **kidneys** clearly going.

It's powerful, but not without care,
Ciprofloxacin—nurses, beware.
With clear instruction, proper scan,
This med can work just like you planned.

METRONIDAZOLE (FLAGYL)

Antibiotic / Antiprotozoal - Nitroimidazole Class

Metronidazole, tough and sly,
Fights the bugs where others die.
An **antibiotic** and **antiprotozoal** mix,
For **anaerobes** and **parasite tricks**.
Treats **C. diff**, **trich**, and **BV**,
Also **H. pylori** in the GI spree.
Giardiasis, **amebiasis**, it's the fix,
And for **pelvic infections**, it's in the mix.

Disrupts the **DNA** of bugs,
So they can't multiply or shrug.
Given **oral**, **IV**, or **topical gel**,
It kills deep where the **anaerobes dwell**.
Side effects you should know:
Nausea, headache, metallic flow.
Sometimes **dark urine** makes a show,
But it's harmless—just let them know.

Can cause **seizures**, **peripheral nerves**,
With **long-term use**, so check those curves.
Also **GI upset, stomatitis**, too—
So monitor closely all the way through.
Black Box Warning loud and bold:
Carcinogenic in rats when told.
So use it only when it's right,
Not as a daily or casual fight.

Alcohol warning—big and clear:
Disulfiram reaction may appear.
Flushing, vomiting, heart racing high—
So **no booze** till 3 days go by.
Check **CBC** if it's used long,
Leukopenia may come along.
Teach about **neuro signs** like tingling feet,
And when to stop or hit repeat.

Metronidazole—stealth and strong,
To right the gut and fight the wrong.
With careful eyes and nurse-led talk,
You'll guide each dose like a med-wise hawk

MEROPENEM
Antibiotic - Carbapenem (Broad-Spectrum Beta-Lactam)

Meropenem, a mighty name,
A **broad-spectrum** drug in the **carbapenem** game.
It **kills bacteria cell walls** tight,
By blocking **peptidoglycan** outright.
Used in **severe infections** wide—
Sepsis, meningitis, intra-abdominal tide.
Also great for **skin, lungs,** and **UTI**,
When weaker antibiotics say goodbye.

Given **IV** only—never by mouth,
It works **fast and strong** to head off south.
Dose by **weight** and **renal score**,
Adjust in **kidney failure** or more.
Side effects that nurses scan:
Seizures, especially if they have a **CNS plan**.
Also **rash, N/V,** and **diarrhea**,
And possible signs of **superinfection fear**.

Watch for **anaphylaxis** shock,
Especially in those with a **penicillin block**.
Though rare, a **cross-reaction** can unfold,
So **check allergy history** bold.
No Black Box Warning, but be wise—
Monitor for seizures as they rise.
And if **renal dysfunction** joins the mix,
Toxicity risk may quickly stick.

It **interacts** with **valproic acid**,
Reducing levels—seizures get placid.
So if they're on **Depakote** for control,
Expect to play a backup role.
Teach: **Finish the course**, don't stop too soon,
Even if they feel over the moon.
And watch for signs of **diarrhea** that stinks—
Could be **C. diff**, so think and link.

Meropenem—a last-line shield,
In infection wars, it won't yield.
With **renal checks** and nurse-led care,
This drug defends when others despair.

PIPERACILLIN-TAZOBACTAM (ZOSYN)

Antibiotic – Extended-Spectrum Penicillin + Beta-Lactamase Inhibitor

Piperacillin-Tazobactam, Zosyn's name,
A **combo med** with infection fame.
Piperacillin fights with penicillin power,
While **tazobactam** gives beta-lactamase showers.
Used for **serious infections** bold:
Pneumonia, sepsis, intra-abdominal hold.
Skin, urinary, and more it clears,
Even used in **neutropenic fevers** and fears.
It's given **IV**—no oral form,
In hospitals where bugs swarm.
It works against **gram-negatives**, too,
Like **Pseudomonas**—that tricky crew.
Side effects you'll want to chart:
Diarrhea, nausea, rash may start.
Also **electrolyte shifts** to track,
Like **hypokalemia** sneaking back.
Can cause **anaphylaxis**, quick and loud,
Especially in the **penicillin crowd**.
So check **allergy history** right away,
Before you hang that Zosyn tray.
No Black Box Warning, but don't forget,
This med can still cause **C. diff** threat.
So monitor for **severe GI pain**,
And **watery stool** that won't abstain.

Check **renal labs, BUN**, and **creatinine**,
Since **dose adjustment** may begin.
And **peak/trough levels**? Not routine,
But **timing the doses** keeps it clean.
Can interact with **anticoagulants**, too,
May raise **bleeding risk** in view.
And **aminoglycosides**, if combined,
Need spacing out—watch the line.
Teach: It's IV only, no pills to take,
But tell them why it fights so great.
And if they feel **itchy, short of breath**,
Call the nurse—it could mean death.
Piperacillin-Tazobactam, broad and bold,
A hospital hero when fevers unfold.
With **labs, checks**, and nurse control,
This powerful duo can meet the goal.

VANCOMYCIN (VANCOCIN)
Glycopeptide Antibiotic – Cell Wall Inhibitor

Vancomycin, the heavyweight champ,
Fights **gram-positive bugs** that set up camp.
From **MRSA** to **C. diff spores**,
It kicks down bacterial doors.
Works by halting **cell wall creation**,
A **glycopeptide** in high rotation.
Used in **sepsis**, **pneumonia**, and joint infection,
Even for **endocarditis** protection.
IV for most, but **PO for C. diff**,
It's not absorbed—just local stiff.
So know the route, it's not the same—
Each one plays a different game.
Side effects? Let's start the scan:
First up is the **Red Man**.
Red Man Syndrome—flushing face,
From **infusing too fast**—slow the pace!

Also may cause **nephrotoxicity**,
And **ototoxicity's** possibility.
So monitor **creatinine**, **urine flow**,
And check for **ringing ears** that grow.
Trough levels? Yes! We check them right,
To keep the dose within the light.
Aim for **10–20 mcg/mL** zone,
To hit the bug, not break the bone.
Infuse over 60 minutes, slow,
And through a **central line**, if you know.
Peripheral veins may get inflamed—
So monitor sites and call what's pained.

No Black Box Warning, but it's high-risk,
So double-check your dosing list.
And **rotate sites** if IV stays,
To avoid **phlebitis** in ugly ways.
Teach to **report changes in hearing**,
Or **kidney pain** that starts appearing.
Hydration helps to flush it clear,
And labs are drawn to keep it near.
Vancomycin—a bug's true test,
But needs a **nurse** to give it best.
With **vitals**, **labs**, and steady hand,
You'll guide this med just as planned.

Part VII
GI, Endocrine & Electrolyte Support

DESMOPRESSIN (DDAVP, NOCDURNA, STIMATE)

Synthetic Antidiuretic Hormone (ADH Analog)

Desmopressin comes to play,
When **ADH** has gone away.
It mimics what the **pituitary** gives,
So **fluid balance** finely lives.
It's used for **DI**, the central kind,
Where **urine floods** and thirst won't unwind.
Also treats **bedwetting nights**,
And **bleeding disorders** like **von Willebrand's** fights.

It works on **renal collecting ducts**,
To **hold in water**, no leaks or flux.
It **reduces urine**, raises **volume in blood**,
Helps stop the **electrolyte flood**.
Side effects you must review:
Headache, nausea, facial flush too.
But the most critical red light sign?
Hyponatremia—cross the line.

Watch for **confusion, seizures, bloat**,
Lethargy, or a sluggish note.
Check **sodium, I&O**,
And **daily weights** to catch the flow.
It comes **oral, IV, nasal spray**,
But **nasal route** needs special say:
Can **irritate** or **cause nosebleeds**,
So rotate nares and meet their needs.

Teach them to **limit fluid intake**,
Especially when taking for bladder's sake.

Too much water, not enough salt—
And **seizures** may be the result.
No Black Box Warning, but use wise,
Especially in **young** or **elderly eyes**.
Also avoid in **heart disease**,
Or if **hypertension** starts to tease.

It's small but mighty, works just right,
To **slow down urine** overnight.
With **labs and teaching** close at hand,
Desmopressin takes its stand.

DEXTROSE 50% (D50)
Hypertonic Solution - Glucose Elevating Agent

Dextrose 50, fast and sweet,
For when the **blood sugar tanks** in heat.
A **hypertonic sugar blast**,
To bring them out of low—and fast.
Used in **hypoglycemia severe**,
When **oral glucose** isn't near.
Given **IV push**, it's thick and dense,
To make that **glucose rise immense**.

Unconscious, **seizing**, pale and cold?
This is the **go-to** nurse's gold.
It fuels the brain when sugar's gone,
So consciousness can turn back on.
Side effects are usually mild,
But can become a little wild:
Vein irritation, tissue damage,
Especially if you **miss the passage**.

Can cause **hyperglycemia**, too,
So monitor sugar **before and through**.
Recheck that **BG** 15 out,
To see if you should roundabout.
Must use a **large-bore vein** with care—
Infiltration? Then stop right there.
Extravasation burns like fire,
Can lead to **necrosis** that's dire.

Teach the team: This isn't for fun,
It's for **emergencies**, not just anyone.
Used with **insulin** at times as pair,
To balance highs with thoughtful care.

No Black Box Warning, but tread wise,
It's potent sugar in disguise.
And if **rebound hypoglycemia** hits,
Make sure they eat—**not just quick fix**.

Dextrose 50—bold and bright,
Turns **code brown** into light.
With sharp IVs and steady hand,
You'll help this sugar **take a stand**.

ESOMEPRAZOLE (NEXIUM)

Proton Pump Inhibitor (PPI)

Esomeprazole, a **PPI**,
Stops the **acid** that climbs too high.
It blocks the **H+/K+ ATPase**,
To end that **burning gastric phase**.
Used for **GERD** and **ulcer pain**,
And **H. pylori** in stomach's domain.
Also used for **Zollinger-Ellison** flares,
Where **acid overproduction** tears.

Take it **before meals**, early on,
So acid stays **off** all day long.
It comes **oral** or **IV**, too,
Depending what the patient's going through.
Side effects are mild but true:
Headache, nausea, gas, a few.
But long-term use may raise some flags—
Like **B12 deficiency** or **magnesium lags**.

Risk of **osteoporosis**, too,
From **decreased calcium absorption** through.
May also lead to **C. diff infection**,
So nurse, apply some close inspection.
No **Black Box Warning**, but don't dismiss—
With long-term use, **labs can miss**.
So monitor **Mg**, and watch the bone,
Especially when patients take it alone.

It **interacts** with drugs in kind,
Like **clopidogrel**, which you'll find—
It may **reduce antiplatelet might**,
So review the meds to dose it right.
Teach: **Don't crush** or **chew the pill**,
Swallow whole, as that fits the bill.
And if it's **IV**, give slow and neat,
To **reduce irritation** with that heat.

Esomeprazole—the "purple pill",
That helps the **acid storms stand still**.
With teaching, checks, and nursing grace,
You'll keep the gut a safer place.

FAMOTIDINE (PEPCID)

H2 Receptor Antagonist – Antacid / Antiulcer Agent

Famotidine, stomach's friend,
Helps the **acid overload** suspend.
It blocks **H2 receptors** at the gate,
To keep the **gastric acid** rate down straight.
Used for **GERD, ulcers, heartburn**, too,
And **stress ulcer prophylaxis** in ICU.
It's often used **before surgery**,
To guard against **aspiration injury**.

Given **oral** or **IV line**,
It kicks in fast and works just fine.
Take it **with or without food**,
But at **bedtime** it's especially good.
Side effects? Usually light—
But **headache, dizziness**, may take flight.
Also rare: **arrhythmia, confusion**,
Especially in **elderly infusion**.

It can cause **B12 deficiency**,
If used **long-term** or chronically.
So monitor **labs** and teach with care,
To watch for signs that might be there.
No Black Box Warning, which is great,
But don't assume it's always safe.
Caution in those with **renal decline**,
Adjust the dose to keep it fine.

It **interacts** with very few,
Unlike PPIs—that's good news!
Still tell patients: **No alcohol**,
And avoid food that makes reflux call.
Teach them: **Don't double dose**,
If a dose is missed, wait for the next close.
Report any **black stools, vomiting red**,
These are signs of **bleeding** ahead.

Famotidine—a gentle guard,
That keeps the gut from working hard.
With teaching, checks, and patient trust,
This acid-fighter does what it must.

GLUCAGON (GLUCAGEN)
Antihypoglycemic Agent - Pancreatic Hormone

Glucagon comes when sugar drops,
And oral snacks just hit the stops.
It tells the **liver**: "Time to give—
Release that **glucose** so they live!"
Used in **severe hypoglycemia**,
When **IV dextrose** brings anemia.
Also treats **beta blocker overdose**,
To get the **heart rate** back, not close.

It boosts **glycogen breakdown** quick,
And raises **blood glucose** with one stick.
Given **IM**, **subQ**, or **IV**,
It's **life-saving** when **LOC** is free.
Side effects are mostly tame:
Nausea, **vomiting**, part of the game.
But if they're awake enough to eat,
Then follow up with **carbs** complete.

Watch for signs of **hypokalemia**,
And **BP changes** with anemia.
In **overdose**, it helps the heart—
So **monitor ECG** from the start.
No **Black Box Warning**, but take care:
It won't work if **glycogen's not there**.
In **starvation**, **alcoholics**, or liver disease,
You might not get the sugar release.

Teach the family: **Give, then roll**—
Patient's side, to guard control.
Watch for **vomit** after the med,
And **call for help**—don't go ahead.
After **consciousness** comes back through,
Give **carbs and protein**—follow through.
Prevent another sudden dive,
By helping sugar levels thrive.

Glucagon—a rescue blast,
That helps when sugars crash too fast.
With training, timing, and nurse-led prep,
This tiny shot brings back each step.

INSULIN REGULAR (HUMULIN R, NOVOLIN R)
Short-Acting Insulin - Antidiabetic Agent

Insulin Regular, clear and tight,
Short-acting insulin, given right.
Used for **Type 1**, **Type 2**, or DKA,
And in **hyperkalemia** to shift K+ away.
It's the **only insulin** that goes **IV**,
For **DKA**, that's the key.
But it's also given **subQ** route,
When **mealtime glucose** needs a shout.
Onset: 30 to 60 minutes in.
Peak: 2 to 4, so check then.
Duration: 5 to 8 hours max,
So keep that snack in post-dose tracks.
Side effects? Most common:
Hypoglycemia, if you're not on it.
Sweating, shaky, blurred-out sight,
Tachycardia, or cold at night.

Also may cause **lipodystrophy**,
If you **reuse sites** repeatedly.
Rotate spots, keep tissue safe,
So insulin's absorbed at proper pace.
Check **glucose** before you draw,
And dose per **sliding scale or law**.
In **DKA**, mix it just right,
IV drip, titrate by sight.
Interactions worth your notes:
Beta-blockers can hide the quotes—
No **tachycardia** or **shaky hand**,
But **blood sugar's crashing**, understand.

No Black Box Warning, but still proceed,
With **double checks** before you speed.
Clear before cloudy when you mix,
And follow **orders**, not quick picks.
Teach the patient: carry snacks,
Wear a **bracelet**, watch those tracks.
Signs of lows and when to eat,
How to give that **subQ beat**.
Insulin Regular—fast and pure,
But only safe with nursing cure.
With **monitoring, education,** and time,
You'll dose this med with skill and rhyme.

METOCLOPRAMIDE (REGLAN)

Antiemetic – Dopamine Antagonist / Prokinetic Agent

Metoclopramide, smooths the flow,
When **nausea, vomiting** steal the show.
It **blocks dopamine** in the brain,
So **chemo nausea** feels less pain.
Also helps the **gut to move**,
By boosting **motility** in the groove.
Used in **GERD** and **gastroparesis**,
When the stomach just delays its thesis.
It's given **oral, IV,** or **IM**,
Before **meals** or **chemo** hits again.
But dose with care and time in line—
Too much can cause **movement decline**.
Side effects that lead the list:
Drowsiness, restlessness, can't be missed.
But the one that makes nurses freeze:
Is **EPS** and **tardive dyskinesia** disease.

Black Box Warning loud and clear:
Tardive dyskinesia may appear—
Involuntary face and limb repeats,
And it may **persist**, not leave in weeks.
So **limit duration**—not long-term,
Especially in the **elderly** or those who squirm.
Avoid in **Parkinson's, GI bleeds,**
Or **seizure disorders** with special needs.
Watch for **diarrhea, depression,** too,
It can worsen mental health in view.
And cause **neuroleptic malignant signs**,
With **fever, rigid muscles,** and **vital declines**.
Check for **bowel sounds, hydration state,**
And teach to **report odd movements** late.
Administer slowly if IV push,
Or **hypotension** may start to rush.
Teach: **Avoid alcohol,** watch for **mood,**
And take the med **before their food.**
Don't **crush extended-release tabs—**
And **monitor EPS** with frequent grabs.
Metoclopramide—a helpful guide,
When nausea won't subside.
But used with skill and nursing grace,
To keep those side effects in place.

OMEPRAZOLE (PRILOSEC)
Proton Pump Inhibitor (PPI) - Antiulcer Agent

Omeprazole, a stomach shield,
Blocks the **acid** the parietal cells yield.
A **proton pump inhibitor**, strong and sleek,
Reduces **GERD**, **ulcers**, **heartburn** peak.
It binds to **H⁺/K⁺ ATPase** with pride,
Shuts down **acid secretion** from inside.
Used for **PUD, GERD, Zollinger-Ellison**, too,
And to heal **esophagitis** coming through.

Given **oral**, usually once a day,
Take before meals—that's the way.
Don't **crush** or **chew** delayed-release form,
Or you'll lose the magic in its norm.
Side effects to note on hand:
Headache, nausea, gas, feel bland.
Long-term use brings other tales—
Like **fractures, B12 loss**, and **magnesium fails**.

Also risk for **C. diff colitis**,
Especially in the elderly and **hospitalitis**.
So watch for **diarrhea, fever, cramps**,
And **report if stools** get foul and damp.

No **Black Box Warning**, but don't ignore,
It may affect the gut's good flora score.
Pneumonia risk can rise up, too—
As less acid lets bacteria through.

May **interact** with drugs like **Plavix**,
Reducing its clot-busting tricks.
So check the list when orders start,
And monitor labs to do your part.
Teach: Take on **empty stomach**, first,
And **calcium, magnesium** could be cursed.
Report **bone pain, muscle twitch**,
Or **tingling fingers** that start to itch.

Omeprazole—a reflux fix,
But needs a nurse to guide the mix.
With **timing, teaching**, and mindful scan,
You'll use this med with a steady plan.

OCTREOTIDE (SANDOSTATIN)

Hormone – Somatostatin Analog / Antidiarrheal / Bleeding Control

Octreotide, a mimic strong,
Of **somatostatin** all day long.
It **inhibits hormones**, slows the gut,
And **stops the bleeding** when things cut.
Used for **esophageal variceal bleeds**,
GI tumors, or **hormone-secreting needs**.
Also for **carcinoid syndrome flair**,
When **flushing**, **diarrhea** fills the air.

It **reduces splanchnic blood flow** fast,
So bleeding in the **gut won't last**.
Also blocks **gastrin**, **insulin**, **glucagon**,
To keep the hormone balance on.
SubQ or **IV** is how it's given,
In **ICU** or **clinic**—nurse-driven.
Watch that **blood sugar** go **high or low**,
Since hormones fluctuate as they go.

Side effects you must expect:
Gallstones, **abdominal pain** direct.
Nausea, diarrhea, or the flip,
Bradycardia, QT slip.
Check for **liver function** now and then,
And monitor **glucose** with your pen.
Also note **thyroid labs** may sway,
And **vitamin B12** may drift away.

No Black Box Warning, but don't dismiss—
Its **hormonal shifts** can go amiss.
In long-term use, check **pancreatic track**,
And **GI symptoms** coming back.
Teach the patient: take it right,
Same time daily, morning or night.
And if it's **SubQ**, rotate the site,
To avoid **lumps** and keep it light.

Octreotide—a hormonal ace,
To slow the gut or bleeding pace.
With steady hands and nurse-led cues,
You'll use this med with practiced views.

PANTOPRAZOLE (PROTONIX)

Proton Pump Inhibitor (PPI) - Antiulcer Agent

Pantoprazole, acid's foe,
A **PPI** that works down low.
It blocks the **proton pumps** that feed
Gastric acid the stomach doesn't need.
Used for **GERD, ulcers, erosive pain**,
And healing **esophagus** from acid strain.
Also used in **stress ulcer prevention**,
In ICU care and surgical tension.

Given **oral** or by **IV drip**,
Just don't crush the delayed-release tip.
Best when taken **before a meal**,
So it has time to work and seal.
Side effects? They're mostly light:
Headache, diarrhea, nausea might.
But **long-term use** brings warnings near—
Like **fracture risk** and **low magnesium fear**.

Also lowers **B12** over time,
So watch for **fatigue, neuro signs** that climb.
And be alert to **C. diff infection**,
With long use causing **gut disconnection**.

No Black Box Warning, but don't dismiss
The risks that long-term dosing lists.
It may cause **gastric cancer** in some rats,
So keep it **short-term** if the issue flats.

Can **interact** with drugs like **Plavix**,
Reducing its power to **bust the clots quick**.
So check the list when starting new,
And monitor labs for a clearer view.
Teach: Take it **whole**, and take it **early**,
Not with snacks or sips too burly.
And avoid **alcohol, NSAID blend**,
Unless cleared by the doc in the end.

Pantoprazole—a GI guard,
For reflux pain that's hitting hard.
With **timing, labs**, and nurse insight,
You'll use this PPI just right.

POTASSIUM CHLORIDE (K-DUR, KLOR-CON)

Electrolyte Supplement - Potassium Replacement

Potassium Chloride, vital and pure,
Keeps the **heartbeat strong and sure**.
An **electrolyte** the body needs,
For **nerve conduction** and **muscle leads**.
Used in **hypokalemia's** name,
When **potassium levels** lose the game.
From **diuretics, vomiting**, or **waste**,
We give KCl to replace it with haste.

Comes in forms from **IV** to **oral pill**,
But with **IV**, you must have skill.
Never push it—that's a rule!
Or you could stop a heart in school.
Always dilute when it's in a bag,
And **infuse slowly**—no pressure drag.
Max IV rate? 10 meq per hour,
Unless **central line** is in your power.

Side effects? You'll want to know:
GI upset when taken slow.
Burning veins if IV set,
So watch that site—it's a key threat.
Too much K? The risks are high:
Hyperkalemia—they could die.
Bradycardia, peaked T waves begin,
Then **ventricular arrhythmias** sneak in.

No Black Box Warning, but don't delay—
This med requires **labs each day**.
Check **K levels, renal function**, too,
And watch for signs as they accrue.
Teach: Take with **food** to soothe the gut,
And **don't crush tablets**, keep them shut.
Mix powders well if that's their route,
And use a **full glass**—don't leave doubt.

Potassium Chloride—a must-have tool,
But only safe when you know the rule.
With pumps, labs, and nurse-led grace,
You'll give this med in the safest place.

PREDNISONE

Corticosteroid – Anti-inflammatory / Immunosuppressant

Prednisone, a powerful name,
Brings **inflammation** down to tame.
A **glucocorticoid** through and through,
That calms the storm the body drew.
Used for **asthma**, **RA**, **lupus pain**, **Allergic reactions**, or **Crohn's domain**.
Also treats **autoimmune flare**,
And **organ rejection** in its care.
Oral steroid, strong in might,
Take it in the **morning light**.
Why? To match the **cortisol** wave,
And help the body **adjust and behave**.
Side effects to watch each day:
Hyperglycemia may come to stay.
Weight gain, **fluid**, **mood swings** wide,
And **acne**, **insomnia**, from the inside.

It may cause **osteoporosis** over time,
So monitor **bones** and **calcium line**.
Watch for signs of **infection near**,
As **immune suppression** hides the fear.
Black Box Warning? Not quite,
But the risk is still in sight:
Stopping **suddenly** is the doom—
Adrenal crisis comes in the room.
So always **taper**, never drop,
Or **BP crashes**, systems stop.
And watch for **Cushing's syndrome face**—
Moon cheeks, buffalo hump, slower pace.
Teach: Take with **food** to spare the gut,
And **avoid the crowds** when in a rut.
Monitor **weight**, **BP**, and **mood**,
And track **glucose**—especially food.
Can cause **GI bleed** with NSAID pair,
So use with caution, double care.
And may reduce your **wound repair**,
So healing might be slow out there.
Prednisone—a mighty med,
That tames the fire but must be led
By nurses wise and patients taught—
To use it well and not get caught.

SODIUM POLYSTYRENE SULFONATE (KAYEXALATE)

Potassium-Binding Resin - Hyperkalemia Treatment

When **potassium levels** rise too high, And **heart arrhythmias** threaten the sky, Kayexalate steps in with a resin swap— Binding K⁺ in the gut so levels drop.

It's a **cation exchange resin**, old but known, Trapping **K⁺ in the colon**, excreted alone. It **trades sodium for potassium**, bound, And flushes it out in a **fecal round**.

Given **oral or rectal**, depends on the case, In an acute or maintenance K⁺-lowering race. Takes hours to work—not fast in a storm, So **don't use it solo** in a cardiac form.

Usually paired with **insulin and glucose** at first, When **EKG changes** make things worse. Then Kayexalate clears what's left behind, While IV insulin buys you time.

Watch for **GI upset, nausea**, or **cramp**, And rare but deadly **colon necrosis clamp. Don't give with sorbitol**, that combo can kill— Especially in those with a fragile GI skill.

Constipation, diarrhea, or **electrolyte loss**, Like **low calcium** or **mag**, could come across. Check **sodium levels**—they may go high, And fluid overload in CHF is nigh.

Use **caution in renal** and **GI disease**, And **never give orally** if they can't poop with ease. In **post-op ileus**, obstruction, or bleed— This resin's a no-go, not what they need.

Rectal route is faster, but watch the gut, For signs of damage—don't keep it shut. Frequent stools mean it's starting to work, But don't confuse that with GI quirk.

Teach patients to expect **weird-tasting grit**, And that poop may come with a sandy bit. Hydrate them well if they're able to drink, And keep an eye on their output and stink.

It's not a first-line, not rapid-fire, But when **K⁺ must drop**, and time's not dire, **Kayexalate** can help relieve the strain— Just monitor close for GI pain.

THIAMINE (VITAMIN B1)

Water-Soluble Vitamin - Nutritional Supplement / Neuroprotective Agent

Thiamine, also **Vitamin B1**,
A vital nutrient second to none.
It powers up **glucose metabolism**,
And keeps your **nervous system** in rhythm.
Used in **deficiency**, clear and bright,
Like **Wernicke's encephalopathy**—urgent plight.
In **alcoholics**, it saves the brain,
From **confusion**, **ataxia**, and **memory strain**.

Also used in **beriberi's** case,
Where **muscle weakness** slows the race.
And before **glucose IV** is begun,
Thiamine must go in **first**—Rule One.
Given **oral**, **IM**, or **IV slow**,
Depending how low the levels go.
In emergencies, **IV route** wins—
To guard the brain from nutrient sins.

Side effects are rare but real:
Hypotension, **sweating**, how you feel.
Maybe **rash**, or **anaphylaxis scare**,
But usually, it's safe and fair.
No Black Box Warning, but here's the trick:
Give **before glucose**, and give it quick!
Because if not, you risk the doom
Of worsening **Wernicke's** in that room.

Check **magnesium**, **nutrition**, too,
Since other **B vitamins** may be due.
And in **chronic ETOH** abuse,
It's part of every **banana bag** use.
Teach patients it's not a fix-it pill,
But part of a **recovery** skill.
In diet, it's found in **whole grain bread**,
Legumes, **meats**, and **seeds** widespread.

Thiamine—a vitamin small,
But saves the **brain** from a nasty fall.
With nursing care and timely push,
You'll guard the mind with a vitamin's hush.

Part VIII
Respiratory & Pulmonary Meds

ALBUTEROL (PROVENTIL, VENTOLIN)
Short-Acting Beta-2 Adrenergic Agonist (SABA)

A **rescue med** in a puff of mist,
Bronchodilator high on the list.
Beta-2 receptors it will bind,
To **open airways** fast and kind.
It **relaxes smooth muscle** in the lung,
So breathing ease is quickly won.
For **asthma**, **COPD**, and wheeze,
It brings the lungs a sigh of peace.

But watch for **tremors, shaky hands**,
Tachycardia that sometimes stands,
Headache, nervousness, hypokalemia, too—
All side effects to warn them through.
Teach them it's for **acute distress**,
Not something they should overuse or guess.
Remind to **rinse** to help the throat,
And how to **prime and clean** their little float.

Before and after, take the **vital signs**,
Check **heart rate** and **respiratory lines**.
Use **spacers** for the little ones,
So meds go deep and not just on tongues.
Avoid with **beta blockers** please—
They'll block the lungs and steal the ease.
And **MAOIs** or **TCAs**—
May cause the heart to misbehave.

Black Box Warning? Not today,
But still, don't let them overplay.
Teach **limit use** to two times max,
Or paradox can hit them back.
Assess for **relief** in wheeze and breath,
And signs of **tachycardic stress**.
It's fast, it's first, it saves the game—
Albuterol, remember the name.

IPRATROPIUM (ATROVENT)
Bronchodilator - Anticholinergic (Inhaled)

Ipratropium, smooth and cool,
An **anticholinergic** breathing tool.
It blocks **muscarinic receptors** tight,
To open airways, ease the fight.
Used for **COPD** and **asthma care**,
It keeps the **bronchospasm** rare.
It's **short-acting**, **inhaled** in kind,
And often **combined** with **albuterol** aligned.
It works by **drying secretions** too,
So mucus clears as breath flows through.
It's not for **rescue** on its own—
But helps when used as part of tone.
Side effects are mostly dry:
Dry mouth, **bitter taste**, and **blurry eye**.
Sometimes **cough** or **irritation** flares,
But systemic effects are mostly rare.
No Black Box Warning, but take care
In **glaucoma** and **BPH** out there.
It can **raise intraocular pressure**,
And **block urine flow** in measured measure.
Teach to **rinse the mouth** post-spray,
To keep the **bad taste** far away.
Use with **spacer** if they need,
And clean the parts for better speed.
Works best on a **scheduled plan**,
Not just when symptoms first began.

Onset: 15 minutes—not too fast,
But **lasting 4–6 hours** as it lasts.
Teach the patient: **Don't double puff**,
If one's missed, then that's enough.
And if using **multiple inhalers**, true—
Take **bronchodilator first**, then **steroid** too.
Ipratropium—a team player med,
To help breathe clear and move ahead.
With teaching, checks, and nursing light,
You'll guide this breath med just right.

SUCCINYLCHOLINE (ANECTINE)

Neuromuscular Blocker - Depolarizing Paralytic Agent

Succinylcholine, short and quick,
A **paralytic** that acts real slick.
It mimics **acetylcholine's** vibe,
But keeps the gate in a **frozen tribe**.
Used for **rapid sequence intubation**,
To ease the tube with full relaxation.
It causes **fasciculations** first you'll see,
Then **flaccid paralysis** rapidly.
Onset in 30–60 seconds, true,
But lasts just **4 to 6 minutes** through.
IV only, fast to wear,
Perfect for **quick airway care**.
Side effects? Let's talk deep:
Bradycardia, **hyperkalemia** creep.
Malignant hyperthermia—a rare, fierce sign,
So monitor **temp** and treat on time.

Muscle pain, **jaw tightness**, may come next,
Especially if used in repeated context.
Also risk for **increased ICP**,
So **head injuries**? Use cautiously.
No Black Box Warning, but know the drill—
This med can **kill** if given with ill will.
Contraindicated in burns or crush,
Where **potassium** levels spike too much.
Check for **neuromuscular disease**,
Like **MS** or **ALS**—don't aim to please.
These patients may **hyper-K** fast,
Leading to **cardiac arrest** that won't last.

Always give with **sedation first**,
Because this med won't quench the thirst
For **pain relief** or **mental flight**—
They're paralyzed, but feel the fright.
Have **dantrolene** nearby for the storm,
To treat **MH** and keep them warm.
And monitor closely, every breath,
This med walks close to silent death.
Succinylcholine—quick and bold,
But needs strong hands and nerves of gold.
With nurse-led timing, prep, and poise,
You'll guide this med with skill and voice.

TERBUTALINE (BRETHINE)

Beta-2 Adrenergic Agonist - Bronchodilator / Tocolytic

Terbutaline, a beta-2 call,
Relaxes **bronchioles** most of all.
But it's got a second secret ride—
It calms the **uterus** when contractions slide.
Used in **asthma**, **COPD**, short term fix,
To ease **wheezing**, **tightness**, respiratory tricks.
Also used to **delay preterm labor**,
Though not long-term—just a short favor.
It **stimulates beta-2 receptors** clean,
To **relax smooth muscle** in the scene.
So lungs expand, and uterus chills,
But it comes with **tachycardic thrills**.
Given **SubQ**, **oral**, or **IV**,
Depending where the crisis be.
But OB use is off-label now,
Still done sometimes, but check the how.

Side effects? There's quite a few:
Tachycardia, **palpitations**, too.
Tremor, **nervousness**, and **headache pain**,
Hypokalemia can also reign.
In OB, it can raise a flag:
Pulmonary edema, don't let it lag.
So monitor **lungs**, **I&Os**, and **pulse**,
To avoid a dangerous convulse.
Black Box Warning for OB use—
Oral terbutaline is not the truce.

Shouldn't be used for **more than 48 hours**,
Or it may bring maternal powers
Of **cardiac risk**, **BP fall**,
And complications you must recall.
Teach to report if **heart feels fast**,
Or if they're shaky or can't last.
And if they're using it to breathe,
Teach proper **inhaler** technique with ease.
Terbutaline—a double tool,
But not a med to give by rule.
With **monitoring**, **nurse command**, and care,
You'll use it safely anywhere.

Part IX
Antipsychotics, Antiemetics & Miscellaneous

DROPERIDOL (INAPSINE)
Antiemetic – Butyrophenone / Dopamine (D2) Antagonist

Droperidol—a potent med,
For **nausea**, **vomit**, and heads misled.
Blocks **dopamine** at **D2 spots**,
Calms the gut when it ties in knots.
Used in **post-op** and **chemo care**,
When **nausea** lingers in the air.
Also used for **agitation**,
Or in **procedure sedation** stations.
But here's the thing that's most severe—
A **Black Box Warning** nurses fear:
It can **prolong the QT wave**,
Leading to **torsades**—a rhythm grave.
So get a **baseline ECG**,
And monitor **heart rhythm** carefully.
Avoid in patients with **electrolyte lows**—
Like **hypokalemia**, where danger grows.

Side effects? There's more to name:
Sedation, **dizziness**, not so tame.
Extrapyramidal symptoms may arise—
Like **rigid muscles**, or **rolling eyes**.
It may also drop **BP down**,
So monitor for **hypotension** frown.
And **restlessness** or **anxiety**,
Can sneak in unexpectedly.
No use in Parkinson's disease,
Or in the elderly without ease.
Also avoid with **other QT drugs**,
Like **haloperidol** or **ziprasidone** hugs.

Given **IM or slow IV**,
Push slow—don't make the pressure dive.
It's short and fast, so keep eyes keen,
To keep the rhythm calm and clean.
Teach to rise **slow** after their dose,
As **orthostatic drops** are close.
And report signs of **palpitations**,
Or sudden **faint** in weird situations.
Droperidol—small but bold,
Not for everyone young or old.
With **monitoring sharp**, and knowledge deep,
This antiemetic earns its keep.

GLYCOPYRROLATE (ROBINUL)

Anticholinergic - Antisecretory Agent

Glycopyrrolate, dry and sleek,
It stops the **secretions** that glands leak.
An **anticholinergic** by name and class,
It blocks **acetylcholine**—smooth and fast.
Used before **surgery**, nice and clean,
To keep the **airway dry** and scene serene.
Also used for **peptic ulcers** pain,
And **chronic drooling** some can't restrain.

It reduces **saliva, sweat**, and more,
So airways stay dry at the **intubation door**.
Sometimes used in **palliative care**,
To ease the **"death rattle"** with gentle air.
Side effects come from drying wide—
Dry mouth, blurred vision, can't pee, can't hide.
Also causes **constipation**,
And raises **HR** in some situations.

Unlike some drugs in its zone,
It **doesn't cross the blood-brain dome**.
So **less sedation, no CNS fog**,
Unlike **atropine** or that **scopolamine log**.
Monitor HR, especially fast,
As **tachycardia** may not last.
Caution in **elderly, GI obstruction**,
Or **urinary retention** dysfunction.

No Black Box Warning, but teach with care,
About **heat intolerance** and **sun glare**.
This med blocks **sweating**, raising risk,
For **hyperthermia** in heat that's brisk.
Teach to sip **fluids, sugar-free gum**,
And **rise up slowly**, if feeling numb.
No **alcohol, antihistamines**, stacked on top—
That combo can make their vitals drop.

Glycopyrrolate—subtle but sharp,
A drying med that hits the mark.
With monitoring and mindful prep,
You'll guide each dose with seasoned step.

HALOPERIDOL (HALDOL)

Antipsychotic – First-Generation (Typical), High Potency

Haloperidol, strong and bold,
Treats **psychosis** that takes hold.
A **dopamine blocker** in the brain,
To calm **agitation, hallucinations,** pain.
Used for **schizophrenia, acute delirium,**
And sometimes **Tourette's** or **ICU delirium.**
Also given in **behavioral outbursts,**
When **verbal redirection** doesn't work first.
Blocks D2 receptors with heavy might,
So **EPS** may come to light.
Think **tremors, rigidity, restless legs,**
Or sudden **dystonia** that sharply begs.
Side effects you must know well:
Sedation, orthostatic spell,
Dry mouth, blurred vision, urine retain,
And **prolonged QT** in the cardiac lane.

Black Box Warning stands quite tall:
Increased mortality in elderly call,
Especially those with **dementia psychosis**—
So weigh the risk before the doses.
Also rare but very real,
Is **NMS**—a critical deal:
Neuroleptic Malignant Syndrome shows
With **fever, rigid muscles,** and **vitals that go.**

Check **EKG** before you start,
And monitor that **QT heart.**
It's often given **IM push,**
But **oral tabs** and **depot** also hush.
Depot form—long-acting shot,
Good for those who **meds forgot.**
But watch the **injection site** and track
How long it takes to bring symptoms back.
Teach: **No driving** till they know
How deep the **sedation** goes.
Avoid **alcohol, CNS depressants** too—
This drug brings calm, but not for two.
Haloperidol—tough but fair,
Brings back balance with nurse's care.
With **monitoring, education,** and trust,
You'll dose this med with wisdom and must.

OLANZAPINE (ZYPREXA)
Atypical Antipsychotic - Second Generation

Olanzapine, a mental lift,
Restores the mind with antipsychotic gift.
A **second-gen**, **atypical** class,
To calm the storms that come to pass.
Used for **schizophrenia, bipolar swings**,
Mania, agitation, all these things.
Also helps with **psychotic states**,
When reality twists or fluctuates.
Blocks **dopamine** and **serotonin**, too,
To bring the brain back into view.
Helps **delusions, hallucinations** fade,
While **mood stability** gets remade.
Given **oral**, or **IM shot** on cue,
The **rapid-acting** form can pull them through.
But watch their weight and sugar tide—
This med brings **metabolic slide**.

Side effects? There's quite a range:
Weight gain, drowsiness, lipid change.
Hyperglycemia, diabetes risk,
And **orthostatic hypotension** brisk.
Can cause **anticholinergic flair**:
Dry mouth, constipation, stuffiness there.
And **extrapyramidal symptoms** rare,
But less than first-gens, to be fair.
Black Box Warning alert is real:
For **elderly dementia**—death can steal.
Increased risk of **stroke or death**
When used for those with less mind left.
Monitor **lipids, glucose, BMI**,
And watch for signs of **suicidal cry**.
Also **sedation** may hit strong,
So advise no **driving** all day long.
Teach: Take the med the **same time daily**,
Don't stop cold or skip out gaily.
And watch for signs of **neuroleptic danger**—
Like **NMS**, a deadly stranger.
Olanzapine—a brain-based guide,
For **psych conditions** that won't hide.
With nurse-led care and steady track,
You'll help them find their balance back.

ONDANSETRON (ZOFRAN)

Antiemetic – 5-HT3 (Serotonin) Receptor Antagonist

Ondansetron, the nausea block,
Works before your stomach rocks.
A **serotonin blocker**, 5-HT3,
It stops the urge to **retch and heave**.
Used for **chemo, radiation, post-op time**,
It cuts off **vomiting** in its prime.
Also great for **pregnancy sick**,
Though always dose it **safe and quick**.

Given **oral**, **IV**, **IM**, or **dissolve**,
It's fast and easy to resolve.
Onset in 30 minutes or less,
With peak relief from **gut distress**.
Side effects? A few to track:
Headache, fatigue, and **constipation pack**.
Also **QT prolongation** rare,
So monitor **ECG** with care.

No Black Box Warning, but still take heed—
In cardiac patients, **rhythm read**.
If on **high doses**, or other meds,
That **lengthen QT**, check heart threads.
Check for signs of **serotonin storm**
If taken with other drugs that form—
Like **SSRIs, MAOIs** in line,
That cause **confusion, sweating, tremor sign**.

Teach: Take before the nausea wave,
Like **30 minutes** pre-chemo save.
If dissolving tab, **dry hands touch**,
And **don't chew it**, that's too much.
Safe for kids and moms-to-be,
But **check orders** and **history**.
And always **document relief report**,
So providers have the full support.

Ondansetron—a stomach win,
To help the healing journey begin.
With nurse-led timing and vital check,
You'll guide this med with intellect.

PROCHLORPERAZINE (COMPAZINE)

Antiemetic / Antipsychotic - Phenothiazine Class
(Dopamine Antagonist)

Prochlorperazine, a double deal,
For **nausea** and **psychosis** it helps to heal.
A **phenothiazine**, dopamine block,
Calms the **chemoreceptor trigger dock**.
Used for **severe nausea, vertigo's spin**,
And **psychotic episodes** deep within.
Also helps with **migraine nausea wave**,
And **anxiety**, when calm you crave.
It blocks **dopamine** in the brain,
To ease the **vomit, delusions**, and pain.
Given **oral, IM, IV**, or **rectal**,
The form depends on how they battle.
Side effects? Yes, quite a few:
Sedation, dry mouth, and **blurred view**.
But more serious ones may arise,
Like **EPS** and **dystonia surprise**.
Can cause **akathisia** (can't sit still),
And **Parkinson-like** tremors that chill.
Watch for **tardive dyskinesia**, too—
Lip smacking, tongue flicks out of the blue.
Black Box Warning to proclaim:
In **elderly dementia**, it's not tame.
Increased risk of **death** is shown,
So avoid in this population zone.
Can lower the **seizure threshold** tight,
So caution in patients who seize at night.

Also causes **hypotension**, falls,
So check those **vitals** in the halls.
Photosensitivity may come,
So teach them to **avoid the sun**.
And **anticholinergic effects** are strong—
Like **constipation, urine delay**, and **dry song**.
Teach: Report **muscle stiffness**, fast,
Or **eye-rolling upward** that won't pass.
Avoid **alcohol, driving**, and such,
Till they know how the med will touch.
Prochlorperazine—a tool so wide,
For **nausea, psychosis**, and feelings inside.
But used with care and nurse foresight,
You'll guide each dose exactly right.

PROMETHAZINE (PHENERGAN)

Antiemetic / Antihistamine - Phenothiazine Class

Promethazine, a versatile name,
For **nausea, allergies**, or **motion shame**.
A **phenothiazine**, with histamine block,
And a **dopamine dip** in the vomiting dock.
Used for **N/V, motion sickness**, too,
And **allergic reactions** coming through.
Sometimes used to **sedate** at night,
Before or after a surgery fight.

Blocks H1 receptors, that's the key,
While calming the **CTZ** to keep you free.
Given **oral, IM, IV**, or **rectal**,
But **IV form**? That gets quite special.
Black Box Warning—know it well:
Severe tissue injury it can spell.
IV push can lead to **necrosis**,
So **deep IM** is the preferred process.

Also warned in **under 2**,
For **respiratory depression** that can ensue.
So in kids, use caution wise,
And **never give if apnea's a surprise**.
Side effects you need to see:
Sedation, dizziness, dry mouth spree.
Blurred vision, urinary retention,
And **confusion**—especially in aged dimension.

May cause **EPS**, though not a lot,
Still watch for **tremors, rigid spot**.
And **photosensitivity** is in the mix,
So **sun protection** is a teaching fix.
Teach to avoid **alcohol** and **driving**,
Until they know how well they're thriving.
Take it **with food** to soothe the gut,
And report if they feel mentally "shut."

Promethazine—relief on cue,
But needs a nurse who fully knew.
With safe **routes, timing**, and patient trust,
You'll give this med the way you must.

ZIPRASIDONE (GEODON)

Atypical Antipsychotic - Dopamine & Serotonin Receptor Antagonist

Ziprasidone, brand name **Geodon**,
Calms the mind when thoughts are gone.
A **second-gen antipsychotic** line,
For **schizophrenia, bipolar** climb.
Blocks **dopamine** to stop the spree,
And **serotonin** for mood stability.
Used for **agitation, mania's swing**,
Or voices that harshly start to sing.
PO or **IM**, it goes in quick,
The **IM** form for crises that stick.
Helps when patients feel detached,
But needs a **cardiac monitor matched**.
Black Box Warning comes in fast—
Elderly dementia psychosis won't last.
Risk of **death** is higher there,
So use in seniors? **Handle with care.**
QT prolongation is its flag,
So **EKG** before you let it tag.
Avoid with **other QT drugs** in tow,
Or **torsades de pointes** might start to show.
Side effects to watch each time:
Drowsiness, dizziness, nausea climb.
Can cause **EPS**, though risk is low,
Still watch for **tremors, rigid flow**.
May increase **blood sugar, lipids, weight**,
Though less than others that sedate.
Rare but deadly: **neuroleptic malignant syndrome**,
With **fever, rigidity**—get help soon.
Give **with food** (at least **500 cal**),
To boost absorption—that's the style.
Miss that step and levels fall,
So teach this rule and make it tall.
Teach to rise up slow, **orthostatic risk**,
And avoid **alcohol**—no cocktail mix.
Tell them to report **heart skips, pain**,
Or signs that **mood or thoughts** are strained.
Ziprasidone—a mind made calm,
But needs a nurse with steady palm.
With **labs, teaching**, and close review,
You'll guide this med like experts do.

Part X
Neuromuscular Blockers & Reversal

CISATRACURIUM (NIMBEX)
Neuromuscular Blocker - Non-Depolarizing Agent

Cisatracurium, smooth and sly,
Blocks the nerves so muscles lie.
A **paralytic**, calm and clean,
Used in **surgery** or **vent machine**.
It binds at **acetylcholine's site**,
At the **neuromuscular junction** tight.
It causes **skeletal paralysis** fast,
But **consciousness** and **pain** still last.
Used in **intubation, mechanical vents**,
Or when **ICU sedation** is intense.
Also used in **OR's grip**,
To ease control and surgical trip.
Side effects? Just a few:
Hypotension, flushing, maybe **wheezing**, too.
Histamine release might play a role—
So monitor **BP** and **airway control**.

No sedation, no pain relief—
So pair with **analgesics** for patient peace.
And always monitor **train-of-four**,
To check if muscles still implore.
Watch **electrolytes**, especially **K+**,
Imbalances make the action tough.
And in **renal failure**, it's a go—
This med breaks down in **blood**, not **flow**.
Teach the team: **Patient can't move**,
But still may feel each painful groove.

So always use **sedation deep**,
So they're not trapped in silent grief.
No **Black Box Warning**, but take care,
Airway management must be there.
And never push this drug alone—
Needs full support, or hearts may groan.
Drug interactions you should know:
With **aminoglycosides**, effects may grow.
Also watch with **magnesium, lithium**, too—
They may **potentiate** what Nimbex do.
Smooth, effective, muscle tame,
But use with care—it's not a game.
Cisatracurium, silent and still,
Works with skill, when used with will.

ROCURONIUM (ZEMURON)

Neuromuscular Blocker - Nondepolarizing Paralytic Agent

Rocuronium, calm and deep,
Puts the **skeletal muscles** right to sleep.
A **nondepolarizing agent** true,
Used for **intubation, surgery**, ICU.
It **blocks acetylcholine** at the plate,
So **muscle contractions** dissipate.
No twitch, no tone, no breath in view—
So always have that **airway crew**.
Used in **rapid sequence intubation**,
Or to reduce **ventilator agitation**.
Also in **surgical** settings tight,
To keep the field calm and right.
Given IV, onset is fast,
Works in **1-2 minutes**, effects that last.
Recovery takes a **bit more time**,
So sedation must be in line.

Side effects to monitor near:
Hypotension, bradycardia, may appear.
Also watch for **prolonged blockade**,
Especially if **renal or liver** aid has swayed.
No Black Box Warning, but still beware:
Paralysis without sedation is a nightmare.
So always give with **sedatives first**,
Or you risk trauma that is the worst.
Does not sedate, does not numb,
So patients **feel** if you forget some.
Give with drugs like **propofol**,
Or **midazolam** to comfort all.

No reversal like with succinylcholine's race,
But **Sugammadex** can take its place.
If not on hand, then time must pass,
Let **supportive care** be first class.
Teach your team: it's not for pain,
Just makes the muscles still and plain.
Monitor TOF (train-of-four) for dose,
And **respiratory support** is always close.
Rocuronium—paralysis key,
But only safe with an **airway** guarantee.
With nurse-led prep and mindful grace,
You'll guide this med in the safest space.

SUGAMMADEX
Neuromuscular Blockade Reversal Agent - Selective Relaxant Binding Agent (SRBA)

Sugammadex, reversal's grace,
Brings back movement, face to face.
It wraps up **rocuronium's** might,
And **vecuronium**—blocks their bite.
It's **not an anticholinesterase**,
But traps the drug in a **tight embrace**.
A **selective relaxant binding star**,
That clears the blocker where you are.

Used to reverse **surgical paralysis**,
When the patient needs a breathing status.
IV only, **onset fast**,
In just **3 minutes**, its effects will last.
Side effects are usually mild:
Bradycardia, **hypotension** filed.
But **hypersensitivity** may rarely show—
Anaphylaxis is no-go.

Watch for **nausea**, **pain**, or **headache** vibes,
And monitor for **delayed revive**.
If given too late or at wrong dose,
Paralysis might still hold them close.
No Black Box Warning, but here's the key:
Use only for **aminosteroid NMBs**.
It doesn't reverse **succinylcholine**,
So don't misfire in that zone alone.

Avoid in patients **renal impaired**,
It clears by kidneys—**so be prepared.**
And don't mix with **hormonal birth**,
It may reduce its baby-worth.
Teach the team: it's **not sedation**,
Just **restores neuromuscular function's station**.
So pair with meds to keep them calm,
As waking up may lack that balm.

Sugammadex—a modern gift,
That helps the block begin to lift.
With careful dose and nursing scan,
You'll guide the breath back in your plan.

VECURONIUM (NORCURON)

Neuromuscular Blocker - Nondepolarizing Paralytic Agent

Vecuronium, quiet and clean,
Brings the **muscles** to a frozen scene.
It blocks **acetylcholine's** normal flow,
At the **neuromuscular junction** below.
Used for **intubation**, surgical chill,
And when the vent needs patient still.
Also used in **ICU sedation**,
With deep **paralysis** for intubation.
It **paralyzes**—but won't **sedate**,
So give with **midazolam**—don't wait.
No pain relief, no calming mind,
Just muscle stillness left behind.
IV push or **continuous drip**,
But needs a nurse with a safety grip.
Onset in minutes, **duration** long—
So ventilator care must be strong.

Side effects? Not so wide,
Unless dosing errors coincide.
Can cause **respiratory arrest**,
If given without a sedative guest.
No Black Box Warning, but know the stakes—
Airway control is what it takes.
With **train-of-four monitoring** near,
You'll gauge when it's time to clear.
Reversal? Yes—if you're set:
Sugammadex is your safest bet.
Or **neostigmine**, with atropine flair,
To block the brady side effects there.

Check **renal and hepatic** lanes,
As **organ dysfunction** affects its chains.
And monitor **BP**, **HR**, and tone,
Though movement's gone, they're not alone.
Teach the team: It's nurse-controlled,
Paralysis power, icy cold.
But never skip **comfort meds**,
Or you risk trauma in their heads.
Vecuronium—a silent tide,
That stops the breath but not the ride.
With nurse-led care and full support,
You'll guide this med in the safest court.

Part XI
Fluids, Electrolytes, and ICU-Specific

CALCIUM CHLORIDE
Electrolyte Replacement - Calcium Salt

Calcium Chloride enters quick,
For **emergencies**, it does the trick.
It brings back **calcium** when it's low,
To help **muscles**, **nerves**, and **heartbeats** flow.
Used in **hypocalcemia** fast,
And **cardiac arrest** that doesn't last.
Also for **magnesium overdose**,
And **hyperkalemia**—it's close.

It **raises serum calcium** high,
Helps **stabilize the cardiac line**.
Restores contraction, nerve, and squeeze—
But watch how fast you give it, please.
IV push can be **very caustic**,
So **central lines** are often the fix.
Tissue damage? Big concern—
Extravasation will make it burn.

Side effects? They're pretty wide:
Bradycardia, **arrhythmia**, swelling tide.
Hypotension, **metallic taste**,
Nausea, **warmth**, a flushed-face haste.
Monitor **calcium**, **ECG**,
And watch the site of **IV entry**.
Check for signs of **overcorrection**—
Hypercalcemia's no perfection:
Weakness, confusion, kidney stone,
Can mean too much calcium's grown.

Teach patients not to mix or pour
With meds like **digoxin**—it can floor.
The combo may cause **deadly rhythm**,
So keep that risk in clear decision.
No Black Box Warning, but don't relax—
Calcium Chloride comes with facts.
Use in **crashes**, push with skill,
And watch that **heart** stand calm and still.

CALCIUM GLUCONATE
Electrolyte Replacement – Calcium Salt

When calcium's low and nerves misfire,
Calcium Gluconate lifts them higher.
It's gentler than its chloride twin,
But still gets **vital work** within.
Used for **hypocalcemia** bright,
And **magnesium toxicity** overnight.
Also treats **hyperkalemia's sting**,
Protects the **heart's electrical swing**.

It **restores conduction**, muscle tone,
And **strengthens bones** when they've been prone.
It's also used in **cardiac codes**,
Or when **calcium channels** block the roads.
Side effects? Not always tame—
Bradycardia, low BP, pain at the vein.
Flushing, nausea, or **metallic taste**,
And tissue damage if misplaced.

IV route is slow and safe,
Give through a **large vein** or **central place**.
Watch for **extravasation risk**,
Use with care—it's not a whisk.
Check **calcium levels, heart's wave shape**,
ECG can shift its base.
Look for signs of **hypercalcemia**—
Like **lethargy** or **GI anemia**.

Don't give near **digoxin's track**,
It may cause **arrhythmias to attack**.
Also separate from **phosphates**,
They bind and crash—no calcium gates.
No Black Box Warning, but take your time,
This med still walks a narrow line.
Dilute and push slow, nurse with grace,
Calcium Gluconate holds its place.

FUROSEMIDE (LASIX)
Loop Diuretic - Antihypertensive

Furosemide, the **loop diuretic** king,
Helps the body **drop water** like spring.
It works in the **loop of Henle's bend**,
Where **sodium and chloride reabsorption ends**.
Used in **edema, heart failure, renal strain**,
And **hypertension** when meds don't gain.
It **pulls off fluid**, fast and loud,
To help the lungs breathe deep and proud.

Given **oral** or **IV push**,
But **IV too fast**? You'll get a hush—
Because **ototoxicity** may appear,
With **hearing loss** or **ringing near**.
Side effects you must track:
Hypokalemia hits the pack.
Also **hyponatremia, hypocalcemia** too,
And don't forget the **magnesium** cue.

Dehydration, dizziness, and **low BP**,
So check that **I&O** and **labs closely**.
Monitor **weights** and **lungs that crack**,
And watch **renal function** as it may slack.
Black Box Warning stands to say:
It's a **potent diuretic**, not for play.
Excess can lead to **profound loss**,
So dose with care, and count the cost.

Check potassium before each dose,
And replace it when the numbers ghost.
Also **teach about orthostatic risk**,
To rise up slow, and not too brisk.
Photosensitivity may arise,
So warn of burns from sunny skies.
And avoid late dosing in the night—
Unless you want **bathroom flights**.

Furosemide—a fluid flight,
But nursing makes it safe and right.
With labs, heart sounds, and patient cues,
You'll help this med bring balance through.

HYDROCORTISONE (SOLU-CORTEF)

Corticosteroid - Glucocorticoid & Mineralocorticoid

Hydrocortisone, a steroid blend,
Both **glucocorticoid** and **mineraloid** friend.
It mimics what the **adrenals** make,
To calm the **inflammation quake**.
Used in **adrenal insufficiency**,
Like **Addison's** or **crisis emergency**.
Also helps in **shock, asthma, autoimmune**,
And **inflammation** that flares too soon.
IV, IM, or **PO** route,
It gets the **inflammation out**.
But nursing eyes must clearly see
Its long list of **toxicity**.
Side effects? Here's the load:
Hyperglycemia down the road.
**Fluid retention, BP rise,
Weight gain, moon face, puffy eyes**.

Also risk for **GI bleed**,
So give with **food**, it's what they need.
And watch for signs of **infection masked**,
This drug hides fevers in its task.
Taper slow, don't stop too quick—
Or **adrenal crisis** may make them sick.
Weakness, drop in BP fast—
A cortisol crash that doesn't last.
Black Box Warning? No, not here,
But still, precautions must be clear.
Long-term use? Then watch those bones—
Osteoporosis makes its tones.
Monitor **glucose, electrolytes**, too,
Sodium up, and **K+ falls through**.
Can worsen **CHF, diabetes**, weight—
So dose with care, and titrate great.
Teach to avoid the sick and sore,
Their **immunity's less than before**.
Don't skip doses, carry ID,
A **steroid bracelet** is key, you see.
Hydrocortisone—life-saving aid,
When **hormone balance** starts to fade.
With nursing checks and teaching bright,
You'll guide this med with insight right.

HYPERTONIC SALINE (3% SODIUM CHLORIDE)

Electrolyte Replacement - Hypertonic IV Fluid

Hypertonic Saline, 3% strong,
Pulls the **fluid** where it belongs.
A **sodium boost** that draws inside,
From swollen cells to vessels wide.
Used for **hyponatremia severe**,
Especially when **neuro signs appear**.
Also used to treat **cerebral edema**,
To **decrease ICP** like a trauma redeemer.

It's **hypertonic**, pulls with might,
So give it **slowly**, dose it right.
Always through a **central line**,
To guard the veins and keep them fine.
Side effects? Big ones, friend—
Fluid overload can quickly trend.
Watch for **crackles**, **JVD**,
And **bounding pulse** with **SOB**.

Too much sodium, rising fast?
Can cause **central pontine myelinolysis** blast.
That's **brain cell damage**, locked-in state,
So **raise sodium slow**—never tempt fate.
No Black Box Warning, but danger near,
If given fast, the risk is clear.
Monitor **sodium**, **neuro checks**,
And don't forget **lung sounds** next.

Watch the **serum osmolality**,
And guard against **hypernatremia reality**.
Check **I&Os**, and weigh each day,
To see if fluid shifts your way.
Never mix with other meds in haste,
And flush the line so none go waste.
Not for **routine fluid** care—
This med demands a nurse aware.

Hypertonic Saline—powerful tool,
But only safe with **nursing rule**.
With **labs**, **rate checks**, and steady hand,
You'll help your patient safely stand.

HYPERTONIC SALINE (7.5%)

Hyperosmolar Therapy – Osmotic Agent for Cerebral Edema

When the brain begins to swell, And pressure rises past safe dwell, **7.5% saline** may be the call— To help reduce that cranial sprawl.

It's a **hypertonic, osmotic shift**, That pulls the fluid out real swift. Used in **TBI** or **increased ICP**, To shrink the brain and set it free.

It draws from cells into vasculature wide, Reducing edema from the inside. **Blood pressure may rise** as volume flows, So monitor vitals as the balance goes.

It's not your go-to for hyponatremia mild, This one's for when the brain's gone wild. In **trauma settings**, time is key, And this solution acts rapidly. Give it **IV only**, and check the route— **Peripheral preferred**, but watch for gout. Though less caustic than 23.4, It still needs **caution**— don't ignore.

Monitor sodium every few hours, To keep from unleashing demyelinating powers. A rise that's too fast, beyond 12 per day, Could strip the myelin right away.

Watch for **fluid overload**, or rising BP, And signs of **crackles** or **JVD**. **Pulmonary edema** may follow this tide, If volume shifts too fast inside.

Pair it with **neuro checks**, pupils and tone, And call for help if LOC's blown. Also **watch glucose**, it may fall— Osmotic shifts can trigger it all.

It's not for routine dehydration needs, Or mild confusion or dizzy speeds. Reserve it for those pressure alarms, When **mannitol** fails to work its charms.

Contraindicated in CHF or fluid states high, Or severe renal disease that can't comply. Use with care, this is brain-level gear— Not something to push without neuro near.

So when pressure builds and the brain needs room, And **3% won't cut** through cerebral doom, **7.5% saline** might earn its keep— Just monitor tight and never sleep.

HYPERTONIC SALINE (23.4%)

Hyperosmolar Therapy - Emergency ICP Rescue Agent

When the brain is near the brink, And herniation's the fear you think, **23.4% saline** steps in fast— A **last-line rescue**, not meant to last.
This saline's strong—**six times the norm**, A **hypertonic bullet** in crisis form. It draws fluid from the brain's tight squeeze, To lower pressure and buy you peace.
Used in **neuro ICU** with care, For **refractory ICP** or pre-OR flare. It's not for mild or moderate swell— It's for when the brain's not doing well.
Give it **central line** only—never peripheral, Tissue damage would be **unforgivable**. It's a **vesicant**, caustic, high-alert med, One extravasation could leave them dead.
Dose is small—like **30 mL push**, But don't let its volume rush. Give it slow, with a doc on hand, And be ready for pressure to expand.
Watch BP and sodium rise, Both can spike and traumatize. **Seizures, fluid overload**, and more— Could knock the patient to the floor.
Sodium climbs can cause great harm, Like **central pontine myelin alarm**. Don't let Na⁺ go past **160**, And no faster than **12 per 24**, that's risky.
Check **neuro status** every round, For pupil shifts or reflex down. This is a drug for moments tight— Not drip bags or overnight.

Avoid in **CHF** or **renal crash**, Where fluid overload could backslash. And don't combine with other saline highs— You'll swing too far and risk their lives.
So when brain pressure breaks the scale, And mannitol and 3% both fail, **23.4% saline** earns its place— In the **neuro ICU's final race**.

LABETALOL (TRANDATE, NORMODYNE)

Beta Blocker (Non-selective, with Alpha-1 Blocking)

For **high blood pressure**, both urgent and slow,
Labetalol's here to bring that down low.
It blocks **beta-1** and **beta-2**,
Plus **alpha-1**, so vessels relax too.
Used in the **ER** for a crisis fast,
Or in **pregnancy**—it's often cast.
Preeclampsia, **stroke risk**, it can delay,
Keeps pressure controlled in a powerful way.

It slows down the **heart rate**, helps it **relax**,
And **reduces workload** with dual-type attacks.
But **watch for bradycardia**, fatigue, and gloom—
And **dizziness** when they stand too soon.
Avoid in **asthma**, **COPD**, beware,
Because **beta-2** blockade can mess with air.
Also skip if there's **heart block** around,
Or **shock**, where blood can't get off the ground.

Orthostatic hypotension can make heads spin,
So teach patients slow rise—don't dive right in.
Check **blood glucose** if they're diabetic,
It might **mask low sugar**, which is quite kinetic.

Give **IV slowly**—don't rush that dose,
Too fast and the pressure can drop real close.
Monitor **BP**, **apical pulse**, and more,
Especially in crisis—stay sharp, stay sure.

So **Labetalol**—smooth, both fast and wide,
Blocks **alpha and beta** with powerful pride.
In **hypertensive states**, it stands tall and neat,
But keep patient safety on steady repeat.

MAGNESIUM SULFATE
Electrolyte Replacement & Anticonvulsant

Magnesium Sulfate, a powerful med,
Used when the **mag levels** fall or dread.
It helps in **eclampsia**, to calm the storm,
And keeps the **seizures** from taking form.
It **relaxes muscles**, and slows the brain,
Used in **preterm labor** to stop the strain.
It also helps with **torsades de pointes**,
An arrhythmia with a deadly response.

But monitor closely, don't let it slide—
Toxicity comes if **too much's inside**.
Check **reflexes** first—if they start to fade,
You're in the zone where danger's made.

Watch for:
- **Hypotension**
- **Respiratory depression**
- **Flushing, lethargy**, and **confusion progression**

Calcium gluconate is the antidote,
Keep it on hand when you push that boat.

Use a **pump**—go **slow**, never push it fast,
And always **check labs**, keep levels amassed.
Normal **mag levels** are 1.5 to 2.5,
But in eclampsia, we aim for a higher drive.
It's also used to **relax smooth muscle**,
So in **asthma attacks**, it joins the hustle.
But again—**monitor urine output**, too,
If **less than 30 mL/hr**, it's your cue.

So **Magnesium Sulfate**—a tricky friend,
It helps with **seizures, rhythms**, and things to mend.
But it's one that needs a **watchful eye**,
To prevent a crash or a too-deep sigh.

MANNITOL (BRONCHITOL)

Expectorant - Inhaled Osmotic Agent for Cystic Fibrosis

Bronchitol, the powdered breeze,
Helps the lungs **clear mucus with ease**.
It's **mannitol** in a different light—
Not IV, but **inhaled** just right.
Used in **cystic fibrosis** care,
To help **thin secretions** trapped in there.
It draws **water into airway space**,
To loosen mucus and clear the place.

Given as a **dry powder** dose,
With a **handheld inhaler** up close.
Two test doses done at start,
To check for **bronchospasm of the heart**.
Side effects you should know:
Cough, wheezing, chest tightness flow.
Also risk of **hemoptysis**,
And **bronchospasm** you can't miss.

Contraindicated in those who've bled,
With **massive hemoptysis** or airway dread.
And those with **asthma** need great care,
As it may make them gasp for air.
No Black Box Warning, but take note:
Monitor FEV1 before you promote.
And teach to rinse the mouth when done,
To keep the throat from feeling spun.

Used alongside **chest physiotherapy**,
It boosts the lungs' own cleansing spree.
But not for kids below **age six**,
And not in those with **severe CF mix**.
Teach to stay **hydrated**, too,
To help the mucus move on through.
And report if **coughing blood** appears,
Or breathing worsens over the years.

Bronchitol—a lung assist,
To shake off mucus like a mist.
With **inhaler skill** and nurse insight,
This med supports the airway fight.

METHYLPREDNISOLONE (SOLU-MEDROL)

Corticosteroid - Glucocorticoid (Anti-Inflammatory / Immunosuppressant)

Methylprednisolone, strong and bold,
A **glucocorticoid** the nurses hold.
Reduces **inflammation**, calms the storm,
When the body's swelling past the norm.
Used in **asthma, COPD, MS flare**,
Anaphylaxis, autoimmune care.
Also in **spinal cord injury** days,
To reduce swelling and delay haze.
Given **IV** as **Solu-Medrol**,
Or **oral pills** to take control.
It suppresses **immune response** and pain,
But nurses must **watch every gain**.
Side effects you'll need to track:
Hyperglycemia leads the pack.
Fluid retention, BP climb,
Insomnia, mood swing overtime.
Risk for **infection** runs up high,
Since **WBCs** can't multiply.
Also watch for **GI bleed** signs,
Like **black stools**, or red-streaked lines.
Long-term use can thin the bones,
Cause **osteoporosis** and **fracture zones**.
May lead to **Cushing's syndrome** look—
Moon face, hump, and weight that shook.
Taper slowly, never quick,
Or risk **adrenal crisis** slick.
That's fatigue, drop in BP fast,
So end this steroid with nursing class.

No Black Box Warning, but still beware,
Of **psych effects** like mood not fair.
Delirium, mania, depression crash—
Monitor patients through that flash.
Check **glucose, K+, Na+**, and weight,
And teach to **avoid sick crowds** at the gate.
Take **with food**, and **in the AM**,
To mimic the **body's cortisol exam**.
Methylprednisolone—a powerful ride,
With nursing skill right by its side.
With **labs, teaching**, and thoughtful grace,
You'll use this steroid in the right place.

TETANUS IMMUNE GLOBULIN (TIG)

Passive Immunity - Human-Derived Antitoxin

TIG is short for the long name true:
Tetanus Immune Globulin—it protects you.
Given when **tetanus risk** runs high,
From **dirty wounds**, **rust**, or **needle lie**.
It's **passive immunity**, not a shot to train,
But a **ready-made antibody** for toxin chain.
It **neutralizes tetanospasmin** fast,
So **spasms**, **rigidity** may not last.
Used for **post-exposure prophylaxis** smart,
In wounds with **unknown vax chart**.
Also used for **active tetanus care**,
Alongside antibiotics and ICU air.
IM injection is the route to go,
Given in the **glute** or **thigh** down low.
Dose depends on the reason why—
250 units for clean risk, more if high.

Side effects? Just a few to name:
Injection site pain, **fever flame**.
Maybe **chills**, a **rash**, or rare reaction,
But most folks feel no major action.
No Black Box Warning, but still be wise:
It's made from **human plasma** supplies.
So there's a tiny, screened-out chance,
For **viral transmission**—rare advance.
Watch for **anaphylaxis** signs,
Especially if allergic lines
To **immune globulins** or **IgA**,
Though rare, they still can come your way.
Teach: It's **not a vaccine**, but still key,
It buys the body time to be
Protected till the **Tdap** can train
The immune system for future strain.
So always pair it side-by-side
With **tetanus toxoid**, if not contraindified.
Just use a **different site and syringe**,
So both can work without a fringe.
Tetanus Immune Globulin—short-term shield,
When punctures, burns, or wounds are revealed.
With **nurse foresight** and timing right,
You'll guard the patient through the night.

THANK YOU

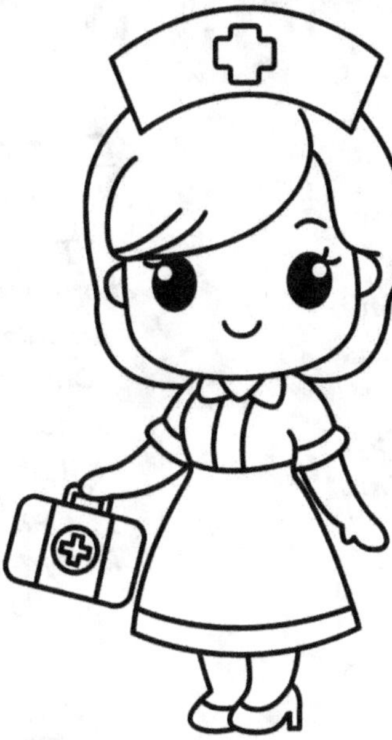

for getting this book and for making it all the way to the end!

Before you go, I wanted to ask you for one small favor. Could you please consider posting a review? Because posting a review is the best and easiest way to support the work of independent authors like me.

Your feedback will help me a ton!

Click **Here** or Scan the QR code below!

OTHER TITLES IN THE
MADE EASY SERIES

Geriatrics Made Easy
Emergency Care Made Easy
Critical Care Made Easy
Human Growth & Development
Maternal & Newborn Made Easy
Mental Health Made Easy
Organic Chemistry Made Easy
General Chemistry Made Easy
Pediatrics Made Easy
Med-Surg Made Easy, Vol 1
Med-Surg Made Easy, Vol 2
Microbiology Made Easy
Nursing Skills & Procedures
Pathophysiology Made Easy
Nursing Assessment Made Easy
Nutrition Made Easy
Anatomy & Physiology Vol 1
Anatomy & Physiology Vol 2

Pharmacology Series
Pharmacology Made Easy Vol 1
Pharmacology Made Easy Vol 2
Pharmacology Made Easy Vol 3
Oncology Meds Made Easy
Cardiac Meds Made Easy
Endocrine Meds Made Easy
Pain Meds Made Easy
GI Meds Made Easy
Respiratory Meds Made Easy
Critical Meds Made Easy
ER/ICU Meds Made Easy
Neuro Meds Made Easy
Psych Meds Made Easy
Pediatric Meds Made Easy
OB/GYN Meds Made Easy

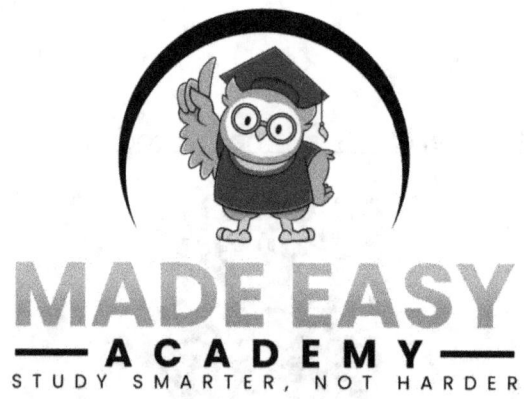